Workbook for Functional Neurorehabilitation Through the Life Span

Workbook for Functional Neurorehabilitation Through the Life Span

Dolores B. Bertoti, MS, PT

with contributions from
Penelope A. Moyers, Ed.D, OTR, FAOTA
Catherine Emery, MS, OTR/L, BCN
Doré Blanchet, MS, OTR/L

F. A. Davis Company • Philadelphia

F. A. Davis Company
1915 Arch Street
Philadelphia, PA 19103
www.fadavis.com

Printed in the United States of America

Last digit indicates print number: 10 9 8 7 6 5 4 3 2 1

Acquisitions Editor: Margaret Biblis
Developmental Editor: Peg Waltner

As new scientific information becomes available through basic and clinical research, recommended treatments and drug therapies undergo changes. The author(s) and publisher have done everything possible to make this book accurate, up to date, and in accord with accepted standards at the time of publication. The author(s), editors, and publisher are not responsible for errors or omissions or for consequences from application of the book, and make no warranty, expressed or implied, in regard to the contents of the book. Any practice described in this book should be applied by the reader in accordance with professional standards of care used in regard to the unique circumstances that may apply in each situation. The reader is advised always to check product information (package inserts) for changes and new information regarding dose and contraindications before administering any drug. Caution is especially urged when using new or infrequently ordered drugs.

ISBN 0-8036-1108-0

This workbook is dedicated to my son Christopher, who was a college student during the creation of this work. He constantly reminded me to keep the student/reader at the center of my focus and always gave me honest feedback and applause every step of the way.

Thanks, Bud.

Introduction and Statement of Purpose

This workbook is a companion to the text *Functional Neurorehabilitation Through the Life Span*, F.A. Davis Company, Philadelphia, 2003. Although intended for use with the main text, the active learning experiences can be used alone or as a laboratory manual in a physical or occupational therapy course on neurorehabilitation. Each workbook chapter presents brief overviews of the key points needed to use this workbook; however, each chapter in this workbook is linked to the information presented in detail in the text, and the text and workbook are used best together. This workbook contains exercises and review questions intended to help the student actively process and integrate the basics of applied neurorehabilitation. Because this workbook is intended to be of maximum assistance to the learners/readers, the authors have chosen to give very detailed answers to the review questions so that these answers can be used as a review of seminal material. It is the authors' belief that learning occurs because of active processing and practice. Enjoy!

Contents

The Role of Occupational and Physical Therapy in Neurorehabilitation

Dolores B. Bertoti, MS, PT
and Penelope A. Moyers, Ed.D, OTR, FAOTA

This chapter serves as a foundation for the workbook; it describes the history of neuroscience and how basic science knowledge and therapeutic advances are codependent. Effective approaches to neurorehabilitation for patients throughout their life span are a common goal of occupational and physical therapists and their assistants, a common ground within the disablement or "enablement" model. Occupational and physical therapy practitioners each possess unique but complementary skills and approaches to patient/client care. This workbook is offered for adoption by both disciplines, to be expanded on by discipline-specific study, which is beyond the scope of this text.

The patient benefits from the skills of both disciplines. It is not only possible but vital for rehabilitation professionals to embrace some common terminology so that patient care is maximized. The principles and guiding concepts presented in the *Guide to Physical Therapist Practice* (APTA, 2001) and the *Guide to Occupational Therapy Practice* (Moyers, 1999) are cornerstones for this workbook. Master therapists and insightful assistants use clinical reasoning and problem solving so that, becoming "tuned-in" practitioners, they can be most effective with their patients (clients).

Active Learning Experiences

Learning Experience One: Disablement Model

Current practice in physical and occupational therapy views the needs of the patient/client through the lens of a disablement model; as a result, the therapy process can address the interrelated variables that affect the quality of life and well-being of the patient and the patient's family. The concept of disablement refers to the impact of pathological conditions on the functioning of body systems, on basic human performance, and on a person's ability to function in necessary, usual, expected, and personally desired roles in society (Jette, 1994; Verbrugge, 1994). The disablement model delineates the consequences of disease and injury rather than focus on only the disease (Table 1–1).

Rehabilitation professionals have accepted a disablement paradigm modified by principles of health as important for enabling patients to remain active within their communities regardless of disease, disability, or risk for these problems (Moyers, 1999). Although there are several different models, all of them focus on the process of disablement or enablement; in other words, they focus on the impact of conditions on function. Some models more than others address the process of remaining healthy despite disability. There are differences between the models, but all possess significant similarities. All models emphasize the importance of function; the word "function" refers broadly to functioning of the body as well as to functioning in activities within specific environments necessary for participation in society (Moyers, 1999; WHO, 2001). Therefore, although physical therapists and occupational therapists may have slightly different ideas about what the word entails, a difference reflective of their respective roles in the therapy process, both professions agree that the patient's ability to function is paramount. This workbook uses terminology based on the broad-

TABLE 1–1	**Disablement Model: Practical Application**		
Pathology/Pathophysiology	Impairment	Functional Limitation Activity Limitation	Disability Participation Restriction
Disease, condition, or disorder, usually consistent with the medical diagnosis.	Typical consequences of disease or pathological processes; loss of or abnormality of physiological, psychological, or anatomical structure or function.	Restriction of the ability to perform at the level of the whole person— a physical action, activity, or task, in an efficient or typically expected manner.	Inability to perform actions, tasks, or activities usually expected in social roles that are customary for the individual within a social-cultural context and physical environment.
Cerebrovascular accident.	Balance deficit.	Frequent falls.	Inability to keep up with peers.

est application of the disablement model and uses terms developed by Nagi: "pathology/pathophysiology," "impairment," "functional limitation," and "disability." Both the American Occupational Therapy Association (AOTA) and the American Physical Therapy Association (APTA) have cited this model, with both organizations stressing the importance of function and the prevention or minimization of functional limitations. AOTA has primarily adopted the International Classification of Functioning, Disability, and Health (ICF) model of the World Health Organization (WHO) (2001) and has adapted it to fit the functional emphasis of occupational therapy, which involves addressing the occupational performance needs of patients through the therapeutic use of meaningful occupations and purposeful activities (AOTA, 2002; Moyers, 1999). The main differences in the two languages is that the new ICF language (WHO, 2001) extends the scope of the old 1980 WHO classification system in a way that allows for positive experiences to be described in addition to the problems associated with disablement. The ICF has "moved away from being a 'consequences of disease' classification (1980 version) to become a 'components of health' classification" (WHO, 2001, p. 4).

Pathology/pathophysiology, synonymous with disease, condition, or disorder, is usually consistent with the medical diagnosis and is identified primarily at the cellular level. Pathology can be the result of many different causes, such as infection, trauma, or degenerative processes. Impairments are the typical consequences of disease or pathological processes; they are further defined as the loss or abnormality of physiological, psychological, or anatomical structure or function. Impairments occur at the tissue, organ, and system level, and signs and symptoms indicate them. Examples of impairments include abnormal muscle strength, range of motion, memory, and vestibular functions. Impairments can be classified as either primary or secondary. Primary impairments are those expected, typical conse-

quences of a pathological process, whereas a secondary impairment is not always typical and may be preventable. An example of a primary impairment for a patient with a peripheral neuropathy in the lower extremity is ankle muscle weakness; a secondary impairment may be a plantarflexion contracture that develops over time secondary to the weakness. Functional limitation is defined as restriction of the ability to perform at the level of the whole person a physical action, activity, or task in an efficient, typically expected, or competent manner. The corresponding ICF terminology is activity limitation. Activity limitation is clearly differentiated from body structure/body function impairments; performance in activities is dependent not only upon the person's body structure/body function but also upon the way in which the task is designed and upon the way in which the environment supports or acts as a barrier to performance (AOTA, 2002).

Thus, it is important to remember that functional limitations are individually experienced, are measured at the person level, and are not to be confused with signs and symptoms of disease. A functional limitation may be inability to remove a coat from a hanger, inability to roll over in bed, or difficulties with dressing, all of which are examples of basic activities of daily living (BADLs). A functional limitation may also involve instrumental activities of daily living (IADLs), such as shopping or using public transportation in order to go to work (AOTA, 2002). Occupational therapy and physical therapy are concerned with some of the same ADLs, while some are of more concern to one profession than to another. For instance, occupational therapy might be more likely to address the use of communication devices, and physical therapy might be more likely to address functional mobility. Disability is defined as the inability to engage in age-specific and gender-specific roles in a particular social context and physical environment (APTA, 2001). Disability is a restricted ability to perform tasks and activities associated with self-care, home management, work, community, and leisure (APTA, 2001). The ICF model (WHO, 2001) refers to disability as participation restrictions; as such, it is combined with the activity component of functioning. Participation focuses on the way in which the contextual factors, either environmental or personal (age, gender, education, marital status, etc.), enable or restrict performance in activity. Both occupational therapists and physical therapists are interested in the interaction of a person's function with the physical environment and social and personal contexts.

Consequently, both the disablement models and the ICF functioning model have always included the concepts of preventing progression toward disability and of promoting maximum functioning. It must be emphasized that these levels of functioning and their corresponding levels of problems are not linear: pathology *does not* automatically produce an impairment, an impairment *does not* necessarily result in a functional limitation (activity limitation), and a functional limitation *may not* lead to a disability (participation restriction). Similarly, focusing in therapy on one problem level, such as primarily emphasizing the impairment level, for those patients/clients with problems in all four levels of disablement may not automatically lead to an improvement in function or in the prevention of a disability (Moyers, 1999). These different emphases in interpreting the levels of disablement do not mean that one profession is more correct in its interpretation than another. On the contrary, the differences are reflective of separate roles in the rehabilitation teams. Instead of the professions being considered duplicative, these different emphases support the need for a close working relationship between the two professions in order to thoroughly solve the problems of functioning in ways that might not be achieved by a single discipline. In general, the focus of rehabilitation professionals is on maximizing an effective interaction between the person, the activity, and the environment, thereby facilitating an "enabling" rather than a "disabling" process. Occupational and physical therapy professionals are arm-in-arm to help their patients strive for the overarching goal of improved function.

The professions of physical and occupational therapy have adopted the disablement and ICF functioning models and their concepts as a cornerstone of clinical reasoning (defined later in this chapter). Both the *Guide to Physical Therapist Practice* (APTA, 1997, 2001) and the *Guide to Occupational Therapy Practice* (Moyers, 1999) were products of the widespread acceptance of the disablement model and focus on functional performance in rehabilitation. Both professions are in agreement with placing their emphasis of intervention on function.

Learning Experience One: Disablement/ICF Terminology

▪ Purpose

This experience will offer the learner the opportunity to practice identifying the difference between pathology, impairment, functional limitation, and disability. Proficiency in identification will lend itself to an easier recognition of the pathology and to increased attention and focus on the more relevant issues of impairment or functional limitation (activity limitation) requiring therapeutic attention, in an effort to prevent a disability (participation restriction).

▪ Materials

None.

▪ Instructions

Using the disablement model and Nagi's classification terms, for the following pathologies give examples of impairments, functional limitations, and disability. The first two—the first pediatric and the second adult—are done as demonstrations. Remember that impairments and functional limitations can be in cognitive, sensory, perceptual, or emotional areas as well as in the physical domain. Also remember that many different types of impairments and functional limitations can be associated with any one pathology, but this learning experience is purposely very broad so that a student can manage it with either an introductory or a more advanced level of prerequisite knowledge in basic sciences and other therapy courses. It is assumed, however, that this workbook is not the first physical or occupational therapy text for the reader; these authors assume some prerequisite knowledge.

Learning Experience Two: Clinical Reasoning and Problem Solving

Clinical reasoning is the process of generating hypotheses, seeking answers, and making collaborative decisions with the patient/client on possible solutions for a clinical dilemma. All professionals involved with a patient use this clinical reasoning process.

Clinical reasoning is a highly specialized cognitive process that includes some level of problem solving. This problem-solving posture requires clinical flexibility so that strategies can be constantly

Application of Disablement Model Terminology

Pathology/ Pathophysiology	Impairment	Functional Limitation (Activity Limitation)	Disability (Participation Restriction)
Down syndrome	Low muscle tone (hypotonia)	Poor scapular stability for upper extremity function needed for handwriting	Failure of school to provide alternatives to handwriting, such as computer use and proper school furniture to improve stability
Parkinson's disease	Tremor	Difficulty with holding an eating utensil	Inability to feed oneself because of a lack of access to adaptive equipment or knowledge of compensatory task procedures to compensate for the tremor
Spinal cord injury			
Mental retardation			
Cerebrovascular accident			
Amputation (upper or lower extremity)			

modified in order to meet the dynamic needs of the patient. Gifted therapists and assistants are often said to have intuition. Some of the skills required in developing effective problem-solving include narrative reasoning, interactive reasoning, pattern recognition, and procedural reasoning.

Narrative reasoning involves learning about the patient's story, in which the therapist then can discern the role occupational performance has played in the person's life. Interactive reasoning takes place during any face-to-face encounter between the treating professional and the patient and the patient's family or caregivers. Information is gleaned by simply talking with the patient and caregivers, starting right at the time of greeting. This type of reasoning gives clinicians a way to gain insight into the patient as a person. There are several different categories of interaction that can be used, including body orientation, activity, eye contact, eye movement, nonverbal behavior, and direct verbal cues including voice elements. Pattern recognition is a problem-solving strategy typically employed in the initial problem identification phase. It is based on the ability to ob-serve and interpret cues. Cues are aspects of the situation that one observes and interprets as potentially significant for understanding the person or the situation. Pattern recognition is this ability to observe a phenomenon, identify significant characteristics (cues), determine whether there is a relation among the cues, and make a comparison or decision. Proficiency in pattern recognition usually accompanies experience. For example, an experienced therapist recognizes the probable impact of a visual deficit, expected to be seen in the new patient referred for functional mobility training after an amputation secondary to diabetes mellitus complications. The therapist not only recognizes but also anticipates common practice patterns. Procedural reasoning is the type of knowledge used when a practitioner applies learned professional or academic knowledge to a clinical problem, often involving knowledge of the human body, medical diagnoses, therapy practice models or theoretical frameworks, therapy interventions, and knowledge from the biological, physical, social, and psychological sciences. Procedural reasoning usually begins with problem identification, but equally important is the ability to then reevaluate the hypothesis in light of new or more complete information.

▪ Purpose

The purpose of this activity is to draw attention to the different types of clinical reasoning used during interaction with a patient/client.

▪ Materials

Materials are needed to successfully enact clinical role playing in both the example and the learning experience scenario: manual wheelchair, eyeglasses.

▪ Instructions

In preparation for doing this active learning role-playing experience, use the following clinical vignette as an example, demonstrating the different types of problem-solving strategies used by therapists in clinical practice. Note the different types of clinical reasoning noted in parentheses throughout this example.

Case Example: One

A 52-year-old woman, Betsy, is visited at home by the therapist and the assistant. The specific referral is for teaching Betsy to perform activities in the kitchen in a safe and energy-conserving manner. Betsy has had a diagnosis of multiple sclerosis (MS) for the past 7 years. Because the specific findings of assessment and functional limitations are not relevant to this particular clinical connection, that information is not detailed here. As the therapist and assistant travel to the home, they discuss the referral information sent by the referring agency, reviewing academic knowledge about the effect MS has on all body systems. The clinicians develop some broad plan for a possible intervention approach (procedural reasoning). Upon arrival, they are greeted by an obese woman in a manual wheelchair who demonstrates an obvious upper-extremity tremor and slurred (dysrhythmic) speech. (pattern recognition: these cues alert the clinicians to coordination difficulties and mobility limitations compounded by obesity) Betsy appears to be delighted to have visitors, engaging readily in social conversation but denying that she requires any professional assistance because her "son's wife comes over daily to fix all of my meals." (interactive reasoning: clinicians gain insight into Betsy's perceived opinion of the therapists' visit, and her socialization attempts may be a ploy to delay attention to the task at hand— the purpose of the therapy visit; she seems to prefer to focus on the professionals as social visitors) The therapist and assistant immediately engage Betsy in conversation about the role of (occupational or physical) therapy and listen carefully to Betsy as she is led into a conversation about her goals, hobbies, interests, and favorite purposeful activities. (narrative reasoning) As the dialogue continues and assessment, intervention planning, and intervention begin, the clinicians continue to use all of the problem-solving strategies as they interact with Betsy. An intervention plan is discussed (narrative reasoning), Betsy's response to the plan is carefully and respectfully assessed (interactive reasoning), and plans for intervention approaches are presented and tried (pattern recognition and procedural reasoning).

This clinical example demonstrates the ongoing nature of clinical reasoning as professionals practice in a problem-solving state of mind, continually tuned into the needs and cues offered by the patient.

Engage in small groups in the following role-playing activity. One person is to be the patient (Bessie), another the clinician, another Bessie's family member (spouse, sibling, or adult child), and the remainder of the group are the observers.

Case Example: Two

Bessie is a 69-year-old white female, presenting to you in the clinic with a medical diagnosis of multiple sclerosis (MS). The following summarizes her functional status:

> Muscle strength: LEs Fair (3); UEs Good (4)
>
> ROM: WFL
>
> Trunk control and Balance: Fair in sitting; Poor in stance
>
> Transfers to and from WC supervision only

> Sensation: Impaired BLEs to touch and pressure; proprioceptive loss
>
> Vision: Requires glasses for correction
>
> Hearing: Nl
>
> Alert and Oriented X3

Bessie is presenting to you today on her last visit before returning home, following a successful short rehabilitation visit for general conditioning after a small exacerbation episode of her MS. She presents "dressed to the nines," wearing fancy, small-heeled pumps with her hair done, make-up on, and wearing no eyeglasses. She is extremely chatty, almost to the point of being euphoric as she prepares to return home. Her family member is dressed in business attire, speaking intermittently on a cell phone. You hear the family member apologizing for missing an appointment. Your task is to review the home program with Bessie and her family member, reviewing recommendations for functioning at home.

Given this scenario, the students role-playing as the patient, clinician, and family member should act out a 10-minute scene, embellishing as desired. Use the example as a model for guidance in identifying the different clinical reasoning strategies employed in clinical practice. Using the following table, identify the different types of clinical reasoning from the clinical example (Betsy). Then, the observers in the case presented (Bessie) are to make notes in the following table, citing examples of the type of information used, cues discerned, and problem-solving strategies used by or recommended for the treating clinician. This exercise can be repeated with more scenarios.

Clinical Reasoning

	Evidence of Interactive Reasoning	Evidence of Pattern Recognition	Cues	Evidence of Procedural Reasoning	Other Problem-Solving Strategies (e.g., narrative reasoning)
Example case one					
Practice case two					

Review Questions

1. What is the difference between the study of neuroscience and the study of applied neurorehabilitation?

2. How do advances in basic science affect the emergence of theoretical intervention approaches in the professions of physical and occupational therapy?

3. How can a physical therapist or an occupational therapist or one of their assistants contribute to the rehabilitation of patients with a neurological impairment? In what way are the contributions to intervention from these two professions different; how are they similar?

4. What is the disablement model, and how do the concepts embodied by the model help with assessment and intervention planning?

5. Define the following terms, and give an example of each: pathophysiology, impairment, functional limitation, disability.

6. What are the *Guide to Physical Therapist Practice* and *Guide to Occupational Therapy Practice,* and what are the purposes of these documents?

7. Describe the value of ongoing problem solving in daily clinical decision making.

_____

_____

_____

_____

8. Give an example of the following: narrative reasoning, interactive reasoning, pattern recognition, procedural reasoning.

_____

_____

_____

_____

2

The Essentials of Neuroanatomy and Neurophysiology: A Neurorehabilitation Application Approach

All students of occupational and physical therapy, as applied neurorehabilitation clinicians, need to master the key elements of neuroanatomy and neurophysiology. For these disciplines, neuroscience is best presented as a systems approach to how the nervous system and all the contributory subsystems control movement. The essential elements of neurophysiology and neuroanatomy are beyond the scope of this workbook; key elements are presented in the companion text or can be found in other sources. An organizational framework helps the student make the connection between location, size, and type of brain damage and how patients/clients may present in the clinic. The ability of the developing, immature, and mature nervous system to recover from damage is complex and fascinating. It is imperative that physical and occupational therapy clinicians be proficient and current in the knowledge of neuroscience and how human movement is controlled and affected by a neurological incident. The reader is referred to the main text for a review of key essentials of neuroanatomy and neurophysiology.

Active Learning Experiences

Learning Experience One: Somatosensory Experience

Somatic sensory information is carried along either of two main pathways carrying sensory (afferent) information to the central nervous system (CNS): the dorsal column/medial lemniscal system or the anterolateral system. These pathways synapse at various levels within the CNS, ensuring the ability to modulate (change) incoming information at every level of the CNS. Although each tract is anatomically separate, there is some redundancy (overlap) of function between the two; this is another example of the CNS ensuring that more than one structure is responsible for a function.

The posterior (or dorsal) white columns carry information about position sense (proprioception), vibration, two-point discrimination, and deep touch. The fibers of this tract enter the spinal cord in the dorsal horn, ascend the spinal cord, and then cross to the other side of the brain at the level of the brain stem, specifically in the medulla. These sensations from the left side of the body, for example, are received and processed on the right side of the brain. Sensory information from all ascending tracts is then processed by the cerebral cortex for discrimination, integration, and association to occur. Centrally, the somatosensory cortex, located in the parietal lobe, is the major processing center for all somatosensory (feelings from or awareness of the body) modalities, marking the beginning of conscious awareness.

■ *Purpose*

The following exercise has been designed to help the learner appreciate the different kinds of information afforded by somatosensation and to allow the learner to practice describing the processing of somatosensation to a patient or patient's family member. This process of "talking the talk" can be a very powerful active learning experience, allowing the student to process this information differently than by simply reading it in a text. Although this example is simplified, it can begin to train new therapists and assistants to be able to explain appropriate neuroanatomical or neurophysiological processes to patients and families.

▪ Materials

Materials needed are a variety of items that can be used to give a cutaneous sensation, such as a sharp tack or pin, cotton, carpet sample, Velcro, and brushes (both soft and coarse).

▪ Instructions

Working in pairs, explore using the different items on each other. The person applying the stimuli to the partner should make sure that all of the following different types of sensory stimuli are applied at different times: sharp, dull, light touch, deep or firm pressure, and two simultaneous points touched. The person receiving the sensation can close his or her eyes, identify the sensation, and articulate to the partner exactly what is allowing him or her to perceive that sensation. For example, one might say, "I am feeling something smooth. This means that the receptors in my skin have received an adequate stimulus to generate several receptor potentials, summing and sending an action potential along an afferent neuron that enters my dorsal horn of my spinal cord. This particular information is traveling within the posterior white column, synapsing on interneurons within the spinal cord at various levels. This sensation is relayed through my thalamus and projected to my somatosensory cortex and association areas, where it is linked to memory of something like a cotton ball [or whatever it is]. I am thus able to identify the object, recognize it as a soothing input and give it a name."

Learning Experience Two: Proprioceptors

The main proprioceptors are the muscle spindle, the Golgi tendon organs, and joint receptors (Fig. 2–1). All of these receptors contribute to overall proprioceptive function, knowledge about one's own body, and knowledge as to its position, static and dynamic. The muscle spindle is a unique receptor, located between the fibers of skeletal muscle, which has both sensory and motor properties. Within this spindle, at either ends of a broadened fuse-shaped center, are muscle fibers called intrafusal muscle fibers (IFMFs). As shown in Figure 2–1, the receptor function of the muscle spindle is provided for by the location of the spindle in parallel alignment with the extrafusal (or skeletal) muscle fibers (EFMFs). As the EFMFs change length, such as during muscle contraction or stretch, the spindle detects this length change and depolarizes the 1a afferent sensory nerve wrapped around it. This 1a nerve also has a critical velocity threshold, meaning that it will detect a length change only if this change exceeds a certain rate, or velocity. If this sensory nerve depolarizes, noting a muscle stretch of a sufficient velocity, it will depolarize and send this impulse into the dorsal horn (where all sensory information enters the spinal cord), where it can connect with other neurons. It makes a direct connection (monosynaptic) to an efferent nerve, an alpha motor neuron (the anterior horn cell), which then transmits a signal back to the same EFMFs, signaling the skeletal muscle to contract. The incoming sensory afferent nerve also makes an additional connection, this time through an interneuron (disynaptic) to another efferent alpha motor neuron, which then transmits a signal to the antagonist muscle, signaling that muscle to relax. The monosynaptic component of this example is also known as the stretch reflex, a simple reflex arc mediated at the spinal cord level, without cerebral influence. We have all experienced having the integrity of this reflex connection tested when a doctor tests it by tapping a reflex hammer on a muscle tendon, typically the patellar tendon, producing the commonly called knee jerk.

Equally important are the functional ramifications of the fact that when an agonist muscle is signaled to contract, its antagonist is signaled to relax. This reciprocal innervation or reciprocal inhibition allows for some of the fluidity in human movement; for example, allowing relaxation of the hamstrings to permit elongation while the quadriceps are being actively recruited to give a forceful kick. This anatomical fact also provides the basis for the rationale behind active stretching, in which a patient/client is asked to actively contract a muscle in order to shut off its antagonist, allowing both active and passive stretching to be effective.

The motor function of the muscle spindle is conceptualized by further study of Figure 2–1. The muscle fibers at either ends of the spindle, the IFMFs, are innervated by gamma efferent nerves, whose cell bodies are located in the ventral or anterior horn of the spinal cord. These gamma cells, however, receive synaptic connections and influences from throughout the human nervous system, such as the cortex, cerebellum, and brain stem. This constant volley of regulatory input onto the IFMFs of the muscle spindle through the collective input onto the gamma nerves sets up a constant resting state of readiness so that skeletal muscle is literally on a steady state of alert or arousal for the task demands to be placed on it. This constant state of readiness is called muscle tone; furthermore, it is called normal muscle tone where the inputs onto this system are absent of pathology. Muscle tone is determined by

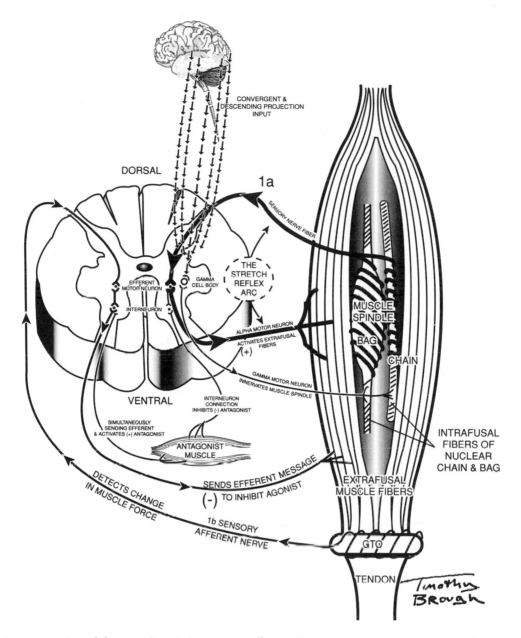

Figure 2–1. A cross-section of the spinal cord shows an 1a afferent fiber originating in a muscle spindle, entering a dorsal root, and making synaptic connection with an alpha motoneuron. The axon of the alpha motoneuron emerges through the ventral root, terminating in the extrafusal muscle fibers. This illustration depicts the stretch reflex as well as reciprocal inhibition. A 1b afferent fiber is seen originating at the Golgi tendon organ, and the connections involved in autogenic inhibition are depicted. The axon of the gamma motoneuron, receiving various inputs, including those from the descending corticospinal tract, terminates in the intrafusal fibers within the muscle spindle. (Adapted from original drawing by Rick Milen, PTA, BS, CP, with permission.)

the level of excitability of the entire pool of motor neurons controlling a muscle, the intrinsic stiffness of the muscle itself, and the level of sensitivity of many different reflexes. The contribution of the muscle spindle is only one piece of the puzzle contributing to the phenomenon called muscle tone. The spindles, however, do play a vital role by providing ongoing feedback to the nervous system about the changing conditions of muscle length.

Golgi tendon organs (GTOs) are located at the musculotendinous junction of skeletal muscle, arranged perpendicularly to the pull of the muscle (see Fig. 2–1). This anatomical location allows for the GTOs constantly to monitor tension and detect fatigue, as a muscle contracts and pulls on its tendon. The afferent nerve from the GTOs, called a 1b afferent nerve, enters the spinal cord dorsal horn. It then synapses with several interneurons (disynaptic or polysynaptic), dispatching several efferent messages, including one to the agonist muscle to be inhibited and another to that muscle's antagonist to be facilitated. This connection allows the GTOs, through the 1b afferents, to mediate nonreciprocal inhibition, also called autogenic inhibition. This autogenic inhibition refers to an inhibitory input to an agonist muscle (the prime mover) and an excitatory message to the antagonist (opposing) muscle. The 1b interneurons can be either facilitory or inhibitory. Therefore, GTO activation results in a myriad of responses in addition to autogenic inhibition. It was once thought that the inhibition of the agonist muscle was the main function of the GTOs. Although inhibition was the first described function, we now know it is only one of many functions, all basically concerned with detecting tension. The CNS probably relies on the aggregate information provided by a group of GTOs from each muscle to extract information about muscle force. The GTOs, therefore, give important feedback to the CNS.

Autogenic inhibition can be effectively applied to a therapeutic stretching intervention, especially in situations where the patient is extremely anxious about movement due to pain. In this intervention, called "hold-relax", the limb is held by the therapist or assistant at the end of the agonist range (the hamstrings, for example), and the patient is asked to perform an isometric "holding" contraction. After the ensuing relaxation of the agonist, the therapist or assistant can then move the limb further into the newly achieved range.

▪ Purpose

The purpose of this learning experience is to act out some of the neuroanatomical connections depicted in Figure 2–1: the monosynaptic stretch reflex, reciprocal inhibition, autogenic inhibition, and the mechanisms involved in normal and abnormal muscle tone.

▪ Materials

Reflex hammer.

▪ Instructions

Working in pairs, one partner is seated at the edge of a plinth so that his or her foot is off the ground, hip and knee flexed comfortably. The other partner uses the reflex hammer to elicit the stretch reflex (knee jerk) in the quadriceps muscle. The most important part of this lesson is for one partner to be able to

explain to the other the mechanism involved, including the monosynaptic stretch reflex, reciprocal innervation, and a beginning understanding of the basis for normal muscle tone. It is also valuable to be able to explain these mechanisms not only in terminology appropriate for a fellow therapy student but also for a child to understand. Figure 2–1 can be used to illustrate the mechanism involved and to graphically guide the discussion.

One partner is then instructed to close his or her eyes. The other partner moves the partner's arm into a new position and asks the person to hold it there momentarily. Then the person moves his or her arm back to a position of rest and is instructed to duplicate the arm position into which it had been moved. Discussion can then follow about the value of proprioception and intact kinesthesia.

Learning Experience Three: Associated Reactions

Raimiste's phenomenon is an example of an associated reaction where resistance applied to abduction or adduction on the uninvolved side of the body will cause a similar response in the involved side. Patients with CNS damage, especially following a cerebrovascular accident (CVA), will often demonstrate this phenomenon. In the patient with a flaccid paralysis in the acute stage post stroke, this phenomenon can actually be very useful in eliciting the beginning of active movement awareness on the involved side by resisting a movement from the patient's uninvolved side.

▪ Purpose

Experiencing this phenomenon illustrates for students the vast interconnections within the CNS. This example demonstrates that a physical input to one body side can have a visible, direct effect on the opposite side. It helps students to recognize the potential of therapeutic touch.

▪ Materials

None.

▪ Instructions

Divide the group into sets of partners. One partner is to lie supine on the floor, with lower extremities relaxed and positioned in extension and slight adduction. The other partner now resists hip abduction on one side while observing the other lower extremity. Remember that this response will probably be very subtle in you, an unimpaired individual with a normally functioning CNS. Discuss the following:

What do you observe?

_____

_____

How can this effect be useful or not useful in intervention?

_____

_____

How can this effect be increased, if desired?

_____

_____

How would you progress this patient?

_____

_____

What did the partner feel who was experiencing this phenomenon?

_____

_____

Review Questions

1. What is the overall organization of the nervous system, both anatomically and physiologically?

_____

_____

_____

_____

2. What are the meanings of the following terms: neuron, axon, dendrite, myelin, neuroglial cells, synapse?

_____

_____

_____

_____

3. How does the CNS send signals, utilizing the following physiological processes in order to transduce and communicate a signal: action potential, generator potential, receptor potential, threshold, excitatory and inhibitory postsynaptic potential, summation?

_____

_____

_____

_____

4. How did the human nervous system evolve? What are the clinical implications of this evolution?

_____

_____

_____

_____

5. How does the human nervous system develop? What are the clinical implications of this development?

_____

_____

_____

_____

6. What are the major neuroanatomical components of the nervous system? What are their main functions?

_____

_____

_____

_____

7. What is a likely clinical picture accompanying damage to the following lobes of the brain: frontal, including prefrontal, parietal, temporal, occipital?

_____

_____

_____

_____

8. Generally describe the behaviors frequently attributed to right and left hemisphere brain functions.

_____

_____

_____

_____

9. How do the receptors function? What are the differences between exteroceptors, interoceptors, and proprioceptors?

_____

_____

_____

_____

10. Explain the motor and sensory components of muscle spindle function.

_____

_____

_____

_____

11. What are the structures and the functions of the meninges, ventricles, and cerebrospinal fluid?

_____

_____

_____

_____

12. What are the main arteries of cerebral circulation? What is the Circle of Willis?

_____

_____

_____

_____

13. What are the common clinical manifestations of a CVA affecting the main cerebral arteries (anterior, middle, posterior)?

_____

_____

_____

_____

14. Explain the following types of lesions: focal, multifocal, diffuse. Describe the clinical implications of these types of lesions.

_____

_____

_____

_____

15. Explain in detail the common signs and symptoms of neurological damage affecting movement control: weakness, abnormal muscle tone, flaccidity, hypotonia, spasticity, rigidity, dystonia, tremor, signs of incoordination.

_____

_____

_____

_____

16. Highlight the different theories regarding recovery of function.

_____

_____

_____

_____

17. What are the main differences between developmental and adult neuroplasticity?

_____

_____

_____

_____

A Life Span Approach to the Systems That Produce Human Movement

Movement production and postural control are made possible by a complex interplay of many subsystems that develop, mature, and age during an individual's lifetime. The multidimensionality of human movement required during different tasks within varying environments involves a complex set of processes that require successful integration. A person must rely on input from several different systems in order to move effectively. Somatosensory information is gathered from receptors in the skin, muscles, and joints about the position and motion of the body. Visual information gives feedback about the changing environment; the vestibulo-ocular reflex is one of many mechanisms that helps to keep the visual image focused during head and body motion. The vestibular system detects position and motion of the head in space, subconsciously helping the body to discriminate whole body movement from movement of the surrounding environment (Sherlock, 1996). The motor system enacts the movement but only as constantly refined and modulated by feedback received from the individual and the environment.

An appreciation of the systems as dynamic, developmentally changing subsystems offers the therapist and assistant a broad perspective on the movement problems encountered by patients/clients of any age. Effective assessment and intervention require that the clinician view each patient as presenting with a dynamic set of subsystems, each of which may present at different points within a unique developmental timeline. It is important to remember that an individual approaches a movement task within a specific environment, calling forth the contributions from several subsystems—the nervous system, somatosensory system, visual system, vestibular system, motor system, and musculoskeletal system—at varying stages of maturation or aging or compromised by pathology.

Active Learning Experiences

Learning Experience One: Visual Fields

The visual field (Fig. 3–1) is the extent of space seen by one eye. The image seen by an eye is inverted when projected onto the retina, so that the left visual field is imaged on the right side of the retina, and the right visual field is imaged on the left side of the retina (Bear et al, 2001). The central visual pathway includes the optic nerve, optic chiasm, optic tract, lateral geniculate body of the diencephalon, superior colliculus within the midbrain, optic radiations, and visual cortex of the cerebrum. Like other sensory systems, the pathway of the visual system decussates (crosses) so that information from the left visual field is projected to the right visual cortex. The optic nerves from each eye combine to form the optic chiasm, which lies at the base of the brain near the pituitary gland. At the optic chiasm, axons originating from the nasal portions (adjacent to the nose) of both retinas cross, whereas those from the temporal portions (adjacent to the temple) do not. Because the fibers from the nasal portion of the left retina cross to the right side at the optic chiasm, all the information from this left half of the visual field is directed to the right side of the brain. The left visual hemifield (half of one eye's visual field) is therefore "viewed" by the right hemisphere, and the right visual hemifield is "viewed" by the left hemisphere.

■ *Purpose*

This learning experience is an opportunity to examine how the eyes see an object within the field of

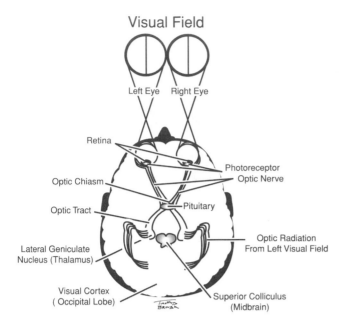

Figure 3–1. Key elements of the visual system, emphasizing the following functional anatomical components of the visual system as a major subsystem of the human movement system: eye including retina, optic nerve, optic tract, optic chiasm, lateral geniculate body of the diencephalon (thalamus), and the primary visual cortex in the occipital lobe. The temporal and nasal regions of the visual fields are also depicted, showing the paths of the afferent axons from these retinal regions to the brain.

Learning Experience Two: Clinical Significance of Developmental Changes in the Systems That Contribute to the Production of Human Movement

The systems approach to studying human movement describes the overall movement system as made up of several subsystems that develop, mature, and age over the life of the individual. Movement is a product of the contributions of many vision and to discuss the implications of what is meant by a visual field.

▪ Materials

A penny.

▪ Instructions

Close your left eye. Hold a penny outstretched in your hand in front of you, at the middle of your visual focus area. Move the penny to the far right until it disappears; to the far left until it disappears; repeating this process also as you move the penny up, then down. The extent of space within which you can see the penny is your visual field.

Find a partner. One of the pair is to present as a person with a hemiplegia post–cerebrovascular accident. The other is the therapist or assistant. Draw a figure depicting the visual field deficit of homonymous hemianopsia. See Figure 3–2 for a clinical insight into this impairment. The therapist/assistant demonstrates to the patient how this visual deficit affects perception and mobility and suggests compensation strategies.

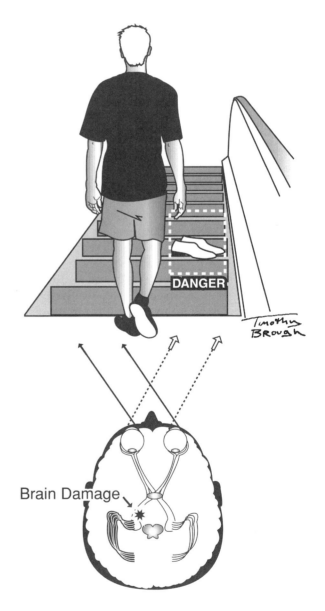

Figure 3–2. The functional significance of homonymous hemianopsia, in this case accompanying a left hemiplegia.

systems working together within their own maturational level in order to produce movement tailored for that particular individual, at that particular time, within that unique environment, in order to perform a specific task. The movement system is made up of contributing systems that are capable of incredible change and adaptation. An understanding of these mechanisms offers a framework within which therapists and assistants can view patient pathophysiology, possible subsequent impairments, and available movement solutions. More importantly, this perspective helps the clinician to appreciate the individual's functional capabilities and limitations and the potential effects of rehabilitation and recovery. This perspective increases clinical effectiveness whereby therapists and assistants can treat patients/clients at whatever life stage and in whatever environment they present.

■ *Purpose*

This learning experience offers the opportunity to study and discuss how a life-span approach to study of each movement subsystem affects clinical intervention effectiveness. If the learner understands the value of age-related development of the major systems that contribute to the control of the movement system, intervention attempts can be tailored appropriately for each individual.

■ *Materials*

None.

■ *Instructions*

Complete the following six two-part tables. Study Part 1 of each table that is completed and discuss in small groups or pairs. Use Part 2 of the table to fill in that information in your own words and then to describe how that knowledge will be useful to you as a clinician working with patients. It is suggested that a pair of students take each table, discuss implications for therapists or assistants treating a patient within each age stage, complete each table, and then discuss all the tables as a group.

Learning Experience Three: Development as a Unique Characteristic of the Individual

■ *Purpose*

As an extension of the prior learning experience, this exercise offers the learner an opportunity to integrate knowledge of the life-span changes of each subsystem into a composite so that an individual will be viewed as presenting to the clinician a unique developmental set of subsystems working together.

■ *Materials*

None.

■ *Instructions*

Create the summary table on page 36, summarizing the salient issues relevant to the subsystems for the main age stages. This exercise is an opportunity to view the typical individual of a specific age stage and at the typical developmental level of the many subsystems that contribute to movement control.

Part 1: Nervous System Changes Through the Life Span: Functional Implications

Developmental Phase	Major Changes	Functional Implications	Rehabilitation Implications
Early Development	• CNS overgrowth with subsequent regressive processes • Axon, dendritic formation and growth • Cell proliferation and migration • Synapse formation • Regional differentiation • Myelination of sensory and motor nerve fibers and cranial nerves; beginning myelination of tracts	• Beginning sensory-motor matching allows for first fetal movements, predominantly reflex in nature • Sensory and motor tracts myelinate first; myelination in a caudal to cephalic order • Areas of CNS to be used first, such as brain stem and cranial nerves allowing for sucking and swallowing, are myelinated first	• Abnormalities in cell migration can result in seizure disorders • Poor prenatal nutrition results in decreased myelination, decreased number of synapses, and limited dendritic branching • Neural connections and maturation highly dependent on use of pathway

(Continued)

Develop-mental Phase	Major Changes	Functional Implications	Rehabilitation Implications
Maturation (Infancy and Childhood)	• By the end of the first postnatal month, evidence of myelination in cerebral hemispheres • Corticospinal tract myelinated by end of year 1, sensory tracts by age 2 years; frontal and parietal lobes by birth, occipital lobes soon after temporal and frontal lobes during first year • Neuronal growth and maturation • Increasing complexity of neuronal processes	• Function is highly dependent on postnatal sensory and motor experiences • Myelination and CNS development closely match Piaget's cognitive stages • Myelination and development of parietal, occipital, and temporal lobes related to development of visuosensorimotor functions; those of frontal lobes are related to motor and emotional development • Critical period for growth is birth to 2 years; areas of brain growth coincide with developmental maturation	• Neural maturation highly dependent on use of pathway • "Growing into deficit" may appear to be the case where deficits are displayed during subsequent development when the behavior or lack of functional ability becomes observable
Maturation (Adolescence)	• Contained brain growth until age 12–15 years; critical growth periods age 6–8, 10–12, and 18 years • Increased complexity of fiber systems and increased conduction velocity • Continued myelination but at a slower rate	• Motor control becomes more automatic • Motor skills attain maximum precision by age 18–21 years	• Competence and individual ability highly dependent on innate abilities, motivation, and practice
Maturity (Adulthood)	• Continued myelination of association areas • Continued synaptic remodeling and growth • Declining nerve conduction velocities after age 30 years • Beginning decline in brain weight and volume	• IQ peaks between age 20–30 years • Learning continues to be maximized because of ongoing development of association areas • Reaction time peaks between age 20–60 years • First areas to show neuronal loss and shrinkage are sensory and motor cortexes and hippocampus	• Built-in redundancy offers great implications for recovery • Plasticity in adulthood highly dependent on use, which increases synaptic strength and efficiency • Beginning decline in short-term memory
Aging (Older Adult)	• Continued growth of dendrites into old age • Decrease in number of neurons; shrinkage of neurons, especially in higher-order association areas • Decrease in temporal and frontal lobe volume • Decrease in size of brain stem and cerebellum • Myelin loss with consequent slowed conduction velocity and slowed neuronal processing	• Higher-level cognitive functioning declines and memory deficits increase • Reaction time decreased, reflex responses slowed, acuity of senses decreased, and motor performance diminished • Basic intellectual ability maintained until at least age 75 years	• Learning continues to be possible well into old age • Due to maintained plasticity, functional decline not evident until critical threshold of cell loss/shrinkage is crossed • Acquisition of new information and conversion of new information from working memory to long-term memory significantly declines • Balance problems • "Use it or lose it"

Source: Information compiled from multiple sources. See main text for details and references.

Part 2: Nervous System Changes Through the Life Span: Implications for Therapists and Assistants

Developmental Phase	Major Changes	Functional Implications	Rehabilitation Implications	How will I use this knowledge as a therapist or assistant treating patients/clients of this age?
Maturation (Infancy and Childhood)				
Maturation (Adolescence)				
Maturity (Adulthood)				
Aging (Older Adult)				

Part 1: Somatosensory System Changes Through the Life Span: Functional Implications

Developmental Phase	Major Changes	Functional Implications	Rehabilitation Implications
Early Development	• First sensory system to develop in utero • Proprioceptors well developed by mid-fetal life • Somatosensory pathways completely myelinated by birth	• Ability to respond to touch first seen around mouth by 7 weeks gestation	• Infant is born prepared to receive and transmit somatosensory information, highlighting the importance of early touch and attachment
Maturation (Infancy and Childhood)	• Most mature system for first few months of life • Conduction velocities increase, myelination continues rapidly, synapses increase in efficiency • Proprioceptive pathways highly developed in early childhood	• Early tactile input crucial for survival behaviors, sociability, and emotional attachment in early infancy • Interaction with world produces physiological changes in neuronal structure and efficiency • Receptor fields narrow as touch becomes increasingly discriminative • Somatosensory information integrates with vestibular and visual information, contributing to beginning sensorimotor mastery	• Early intervention stimulation activities need to emphasize motor and sensory experiences; sensory experience does not "drive" motor ability: sensory and motor development are intertwined • Integration of somatosensory information with other sensory modalities develops the ability to plan motor action and move about in space, called "praxis"; difficulty with this ability can result in developmental **dyspraxia**
Maturation (Adolescence)	• Myelination continues • Maturation and integration of somatosensory processing continue	• Maturing sensory abilities contribute to refinement of skill and emerging body image • Somatosensory system keenest in late adolescence	• Integration of somatosensory information contributes to development of an intact body image • Lack of experience and exposure to novel opportunities limits skill refinement
Maturity (Adulthood)	• Small, almost imperceptible changes not noticeable until after age 40 years • Skin changes, such as dryness and decreased elasticity, affect precision of cutaneous receptors	• Reaction time decreased	• Knowledge based on experience makes up for any minimal sensory and motor decline, minimizing any functional impact • Clinicians can maximize rehabilitation at this life stage by choosing tasks from the patient's past experience and knowledge repertoire
Aging (Older Adult)	• Number of receptors decreased, structural distortion of receptors, proprioceptor atrophy, and weakening of impulse conduction • Skin changes, such as wrinkling and increased toughness, and changes in hair distribution affect accuracy of reception	• Tactile sensitivity decreases, especially fine touch, pressure, and vibration sense, predominately in fingertips, palms, and lower extremities • Decrease in feedback to CNS secondary to proprioception loss, contributing to movement inaccuracies, instability, incoordination, gait disturbances, and falls	• High incidence of peripheral neuropathy • Need to compensate with additional sensory or external cues • Need to make purposeful, more deliberate movement

Source: Information compiled from multiple sources. See main text for details and references.

Part 2: Somatosensory System Changes Through the Life Span: Implications for Therapists and Assistants

Developmental Phase	Major Changes	Functional Implications	Rehabilitation Implications	How will I use this knowledge as a therapist or assistant treating patients/clients of this age?
Maturation (Infancy and Childhood)				
Maturation (Adolescence)				
Maturity (Adulthood)				
Aging (Older Adult)				

Part 1: Visual System Changes Through the Life Span: Functional Implications

Developmental Phase	Major Changes	Functional Implications	Rehabilitation Implications
Early Development	• Eye formed by 4 weeks gestation • Neurons in occipital cortex are arranged in columns by birth, ready to receive visual input	• Fetus demonstrates reflexive eye blinking by 6 weeks gestation	
Maturation (Infancy and Childhood)	• Central visual pathways, including thalamic connections, develop early • Adult levels of visual acuity (20/20) attained by end of first year • Binocular vision (for depth) matures between 3–5 months of age	• Newborns prefer patterns and can focus on objects 7–9 inches from face, such as a parent's face • Infants see initially in black and white; full color vision present by 4 months of age • Young infants can fixate, converge, and track by 2 months of age • Head and antigravity postural control promotes visual development • Postural control subserves visual interest • Depth perception in place by time infant learns to creep • Development of postural control highly dependent on vision through age 6 years	• Neonatal stimulation and parent education programs should include guiding parents in how to best visually stimulate the newborn, including how to arrange an appropriately stimulating nursery environment • Movement and visual development are subservient to each other • Early intervention programming should reinforce the connection between vision and motor development in infants and young children
Maturation (Adolescence)	• Maturation and processing increase • Adult levels of depth perception attained by age 12 years • Eyesight sharpest at age 20 years	• Sensory abilities and motor skill continue to contribute to advanced capabilities, allowing for success with sports and leisure activities	• An age of tremendous opportunity for motor learning and reeducation
Maturity (Adulthood)	• Visual acuity continues to improve during 20s and 30s • At age 45 years, a tendency for presbyopia, caused by age-related inability of lens to change its curvature • Lens elasticity and transparency decrease • Incidence of cataract formation increases after age 30 years	• Sharp decline after age 40 years in ability to adapt quickly to change from light to dark environment	• Difficulty with reading small print and adapting quickly to lighting between environments are issues for clinician to be aware of with patient instruction
Aging (Older Adult)	• Eye structure changes so that less light is transmitted to the retina, and pupil size decreases • Macular degeneration and cataracts are common • Visual acuity decreases between age 60–80 years; at 80% of normal at age 85 years	• Because less light is transmitted, visual threshold is increased, requiring more light to see • Ability to adapt when moving from a dark to a light environment decreases; incidence of glare is high • Depth perception, contrast sensitivity, and peripheral vision decline	• Significant implications for safety, mobility, and functional independence • Older adults may require additional sensory or external cues, especially when in unfamiliar environments • Approximately 10 % of elderly have undetected eye disease or visual impairment

Source: Information compiled from multiple sources. See main text for details and references.

Part 2: Visual System Changes Through the Life Span: Implications For Therapists and Assistants

Developmental Phase	Major Changes	Functional Implications	Rehabilitation Implications	How will I use this knowledge as a therapist or assistant treating patients/clients of this age?
Maturation (Infancy and Childhood)				
Maturation (Adolescence)				
Maturity (Adulthood)				
Aging (Older Adult)				

Part 1: Vestibular System Changes Through the Life Span: Functional Implications

Developmental Phase	Major Changes	Functional Implications	Rehabilitation Implications
Early Development	• Peripheral receptors formed by 10 weeks gestation • Vestibular system operational in utero, providing information about fetal movement	• Fetus able to show generalized body responses to changes in position, such as head righting • Uterine movement has been linked to later movement competence	• It is reasonable to be concerned about lack or paucity of fetal movement as an indicator of movement dysfunction
Maturation (Infancy and Childhood)	• Completely myelinated at birth, prepared to transmit information regarding movement and gravity • Continuing maturation and sensory integration of this system ongoing throughout childhood	• Equilibrium reactions and the ability to right the body develop as vestibular system matures and becomes integrated with other movement subsystems • Early movement activities are related to development of competence over gravity and postural stability	• Preterm infants have delayed vestibular responses to movement • Infants with vestibular problems demonstrate delays in attainment of motor skills
Maturation (Adolescence)	• Vestibular system continues to mature, with full maturity attained between ages 10–14 years	• Normal maturation and integration contribute to healthy body scheme and gravitational security • Vestibular system coordinates with visual and somatosensory system, contributing to refined static and dynamic balance • Balance performance peaks between ages 9–12 years	• Refinement of this system related to experience and exposure
Maturity (Adulthood)	• Beginning at age 40 years, number of sensory fibers and cells decrease	• No specific significant functional implications	• As with other systems, knowledge and past experience make up for any minimal decline, maximizing rehabilitation potential
Aging (Older Adult)	• Age-related changes include reduction in number of receptor and motor fibers, loss of hair cells • Vestibular nuclei have decreased electrical excitability and deterioration in central processing	• Decline in vestibular abilities contributes to postural control deficits • Incidence of dizziness, vertigo, unsteadiness, and balance disorders increases • Increased threshold for vestibular activation could contribute to increased body sway	• Ability to function adequately decreases in new or unfamiliar environments or where other sensory cues are unpredictable • Falls in the elderly are caused by a constellation of factors, including a decline in vestibular functioning

Source: Information compiled from multiple sources. See main text for details and references.

Part 2: Vestibular System Changes Through the Life Span: Implications for Therapists and Assistants

Developmental Phase	Major Changes	Functional Implications	Rehabilitation Implications	How will I use this knowledge as a therapist or assistant treating patients/clients of this age?
Maturation (Infancy and Childhood)				
Maturation (Adolescence)				
Maturity (Adulthood)				
Aging (Older Adult)				

Part 1: Muscular System Changes Through the Life Span: Functional Implications

Develop-mental Phase	Major Changes	Functional Implications	Rehabilitation Implications
Early Development	• Motor units formed and skeletal muscle mature by 8 weeks • Different fiber types developed by 30 weeks • Number and size of fiber increase during last half of gestation	• First fetal movements seen by 8 weeks	• Lack of fetal movement may be an indicator of future motor problems
Maturation (Infancy and Childhood)	• At birth, most fibers are fast-twitch; slow-twitch develop between ages 1–2 years; adult ratio reached by end of second year • Fourteen-fold increase in fiber number between birth and age 16 years; rapid growth spurt at age 2 years	• Development of slow-twitch fiber type corresponds with developing postural control as mastery over gravity continues to become evident	• Children with delayed attainment of motor skills and poor postural control may never attain the normal adult fiber-type ratio • The value of early intervention and movement stimulation is tremendous
Maturation (Adolescence)	• Greatest strength development occurs between ages 6–18 years • Number of fibers doubles between ages 10–16 years	• Increase in strength is directly related to increase in mass	• Boys have greater strength than girls at all ages
Maturity (Adulthood)	• Fiber numbers continue to increase through age 50 years, after which a decline begins	• Maximum strength begins to peak during 20s, maximal in men between age 30–35, staying constant until 50, 20% loss by age 60 years	• Physically active adults maintain and increase strength • There is considerable variation in strength and endurance among individuals
Aging (Older Adult)	• Senile muscular atrophy occurs due to decrease in fibers, decrease in muscle mass, and decline in number of functional motor units	• Strength and speed of muscle contraction decrease; 50% loss by age 70 years • Rate of decline in muscle strength less in upper extremities than in trunk and lower extremities; this distribution contributes to changes in postural alignment and perhaps causes functional instability • Trunk weakness may contribute to less effective equilibrium reactions	• Degree of atrophy highly variable, dependent on activity level and level of fitness • Strength losses can be minimized with exercise, including moderate weight training • Rehabilitation program success is highly dependent on premorbid fitness level

Source: Information compiled from multiple sources. See main text for details and references.

Part 2: Muscular System Changes Through the Life Span: Implications for Therapists and Assistants

Developmental Phase	Major Changes	Functional Implications	Rehabilitation Implications	How will I use this knowledge as a therapist or assistant treating patients/clients of this age?
Maturation (Infancy and Childhood)				
Maturation (Adolescence)				
Maturity (Adulthood)				
Aging (Older Adult)				

Part 1: Skeletal System Changes Through the Life Span: Functional Implications

Develop-mental Phase	Major Changes	Functional Implications	Rehabilitation Implications
Early Development	• Cartilage model of long bones formed by week 6; primary ossification centers emerge by week 12	• Malleable, cartilaginous skeleton models in response to forces acting upon it	• Confines of uterus limit fetal movement; may result in modeling deformities, such as clubfoot, which respond well to early intervention
Maturation (Infancy and Childhood)	• Epiphysis is an active site of bone formation • Vertebral column responds to gravitational forces by developing secondary lordotic curves in cervical and lumbar areas	• Rotational, angular, and torsional changes to pelvis and lower extremities are in response to movement and muscular forces • Weight bearing promotes bone growth and density • Development of head control in prone leads to development of cervical lordosis; sitting and standing contribute to lumbar lordosis	• Fractures of epiphyseal plate may interfere with bone growth pattern and may result in deformity • Abnormal forces, either from limited movement or excessive force, such as in spasticity, may result in abnormal skeletal development and deformity
Maturation (Adolescence)	• Sudden increase in height and weight produces "growth spurt" lasting 2 years, at 12–13 years for girls, 13–15 years for boys • Skeletal maturity attained when epiphyseal plate closes; complete closure may take up until age 25 years	• Girls demonstrate greater flexibility than boys • Boys tend to make rapid gains in strength throughout adolescence, whereas girls peak at puberty and regress by end of adolescence	• Bone grows before muscle, often contributing to muscular tightness, limited range of motion; basis of common complaint "growing pains" • Stress fractures and avulsion fractures are common • Scoliosis commonly appears during adolescence
Maturity (Adulthood)	• Bone remodeling and increases in density continue • After age 40 years, bone resorption begins to exceed bone replacement • Intervertebral disc becomes more fibrous, less hydrated; vertebral bodies are less dense • Menopause creates a great impetus for bone loss in women	• Changes in density and modeling occur as response to weight bearing and muscular contraction • Due to changes in vertebral column, some shortening in height may become evident	• High incidence of back pain secondary to disc changes • Physical activity, including weight training and weight bearing, contributes to less bone resorption and decreased osteoporosis
Aging (Older Adult)	• Collagen less elastic and slower to respond to stretch changes • Loss of bone mass continues	• Loss in flexibility may contribute to hypokinesis • Declines in strength and flexibility can contribute to poor posture	• Range of motion can be maintained, but stretching needs to be done more slowly • High incidence of osteoporosis and osteoarthritis • Age-related bone loss decreases with physical fitness, including moderate weight training

Source: Information compiled from multiple sources. See main text for details and references.

Part 2: Skeletal System Changes Through the Life Span: Implications for Therapists and Assistants

Developmental Phase	Major Changes	Functional Implications	Rehabilitation Implications	How will I use this knowledge as a therapist or assistant treating patients/clients of this age?
Maturation (Infancy and Childhood)				
Maturation (Adolescence)				
Maturity (Adulthood)				
Aging (Older Adult)				

Summary Table (Learning Experience Three)

Age Stage	Salient Issues Relative to Nervous System Development	Salient Issues Relative to Somatosensory System Development	Salient Issues Relative to Visual System Development	Salient Issues Relative to Vestibular System Development	Salient Issues Relative to Muscular System Development	Salient Issues Relative to Skeletal System Development
Newborn						
One-Year Old						
Pre-school Child						
Adolescent						
Mature Adult						
Older Adult						

Review Questions

1. Describe the relationship between theories, practice models, and intervention concepts.

_____

_____

_____

_____

2. Summarize the history of the evolution of contemporary motor control theory, highlighting the premises of the reflex theory, and hierarchical or neuromaturational theory, and describe how insights and limitations from these theories led to the development of the contemporary dynamic action systems perspective.

_____

_____

_____

_____

3. Describe the main theoretical assumptions underlying the dynamic action systems model of motor control.

_____

_____

_____

_____

4. What is the definition of a systems approach?

_____

_____

_____

_____

5. Describe what is meant by the application of a systems approach to the study of movement and neurorehabilitation.

_____

_____

_____

_____

6. Explain how the systems involved in movement production are dynamic in nature.

_____

_____

_____

_____

7. Define a life span developmental perspective, including differentiating between the following functional divisions: early development, maturation, maturity, aging.

_____

_____

_____

_____

8. Describe in general terms the process of human nervous system development, including describing the processes of neuronal differentiation, cell migration, and myelination.

_____

_____

_____

_____

9. What is the impact of critical periods on functional outcome during development?

_____

_____

_____

_____

10. Describe the major developmental nervous system changes that occur during early development, maturation, maturity, and aging. How can an understanding of these changes affect a clinician's approach to patient care?

_____

_____

_____

_____

11. Describe the major anatomical components of the somatosensory system.

_____

_____

_____

_____

12. How does the overall function of the somatosensory subsystem contribute to the production of movement?

_____

_____

_____

_____

13. Describe the age-related developmental changes of the somatosensory system. How does an understanding of these changes affect a clinician's approach to patient care?

_____

_____

_____

_____

14. Describe the major anatomical components of the visual system and the overall functional contribution of this subsystem to the production of movement.

_____

_____

_____

_____

15. Describe the age-related developmental changes of the visual system. How does an understanding of these changes affect a clinician's approach to patient care?

_____

_____

_____

_____

16. Describe the major anatomical components of the vestibular system and the overall functional contribution of this subsystem to the production of movement.

_____

_____

_____

_____

17. Describe the age-related developmental changes of the vestibular system. How does an understanding of these changes affect a clinician's approach to patient care?

_____

_____

_____

_____

18. Describe the major components of the motor or action system and the overall functional contribution of this subsystem to the production of movement.

_____

_____

_____

_____

19. Describe the age-related developmental changes of the musculoskeletal system. How does an understanding of these changes affect a clinician's approach to patient care?

_____

_____

_____

_____

Life Span Motor Development

Changes in all the subsystems that contribute to the production of human movement influence motor development. Each system (nervous, visual, somatosensory, vestibular, muscular, skeletal, cognitive) interacts with the others within the environment in complex and fascinating ways to effect changes in motor behavior that continue throughout the life span. Movement expression, then, comes about as a result of all of the convergent influences and changes acting on the individual at any point in time as that individual moves to perform a task within a specific environmental context.

Development can be thought of as a change in form and function, where form and function are intertwined (Cech and Martin, 1995; Higgins, 1985). The form a movement takes is largely determined by the function for which it is intended. Simultaneously, the function, which emerges or becomes possible, is largely dependent on the available forms of movement and the developmental phase of the structures. Development is not simply growth. Developmental changes occur through the processes of growth, maturation, adaptation, and learning (Cech and Martin, 1995).

Active Learning Experiences

Learning Experience One: Clinician Sensitivity to Developmental Tasks and Issues

Therapists and assistants working with individuals at different times of the life span need to be sensitive to the main developmental tasks and issues that face an individual at that age. Erikson described the developmental stages that a person goes through to establish personality. He linked each of eight stages to chronological age, with each stage characterized by a conflict between two opposite traits. The eight stages can be summarized as presented in Table 4–1.

■ Purpose

Therapists and assistants working with individuals at different times of the life span should be sensitive to what primary developmental tasks are the main focus at that age stage. For example, an appreciation of the importance of feeling purposeful and worthwhile throughout the adult years, when adults are actively solving the conflict between generativity (being worthwhile) and self-absorption, can sensitize therapists and families to the emotional, difficult issues being faced by an adult with a disability. The purpose of this learning experience is to offer the learner an opportunity to focus on the developmental emotional issues that are typically confronted at various age stages and to discuss the influence that a neurological incident and subsequent change in functional ability may pose to individuals at different times in the life cycle.

■ Materials

None.

■ Instructions

After reviewing Erikson's stages of personality development, discuss the implications with a partner and complete the last column of the table on page 43.

TABLE 4–1	**Erikson's Eight Stages of Personality Development: Implications for Therapists and Assistants**			
Erikson's Psychosocial Stage	Age Stage	Developmental Task	Important Influences	Implications for Therapists and Assistants
Trust vs. mistrust	0–18 m	Attachment; developing trust in self, parents, and world	Involved caregivers with loving interaction	Development of trust allows for interest in world and ability to explore it; very important for infant to feel secure and safe, including while practicing new movement skills
Autonomy vs. shame and doubt	18 m–2/3 y	Developing feeling of control over behavior; realizing that intentions can be acted out; beginning independence and learning of self-control	Supportive parents and caregivers; therapist who is supportive, firm but not threatening	As children become mobile, acting out becomes possible; imitation and modeling of others and supportive parents crucial at this time; caregivers, including therapists, should set reasonable limits
Initiative vs. guilt	2/3 y–6 y	Developing a sense of self and responsibility for one's own actions; initiates own activity; a time when active exploration can be either encouraged or made to produce guilt	Supportive parents, caregivers, and therapists	Children need to be able to make some decisions and exercise some choices regarding activity; activities need to have a purpose and direction; therapist should allow children some amount of choice in activity
Industry vs. inferiority	6–11 y	Developing a sense of self-worth through interaction with peers; works on projects for recognition; develops mastery and competence	Encouraging educational setting and supportive teachers, caregivers, and therapists	Children need to participate in therapy program choices, including goals; children should be allowed to record their own participation and progress and note achievements in competence; therapist can set up incentive programs to reward compliance—remember to accentuate the ability, not the disability
Identity vs. identity diffusion or role confusion	11 y–late adolescence	Developing a strong sense of identity; selecting from among many potential selves	Supportive caregivers and teachers, role models, and peers	Self-esteem and body image are key issues; exploration of available vocational choices occurs
Intimacy vs. isolation	Young adulthood	Developing close relationships with others; intimacy and partnership; working toward establishing a career	Supportive peers, colleagues, family (including spouse and children), society, community	Continuing concern regarding self-esteem and sexuality; some amount of vocational success is important

TABLE 4–1	**Erikson's Eight Stages of Personality Development: Implications for Therapists and Assistants**			
Erikson's Psychosocial Stage	Age Stage	Developmental Task	Important Influences	Implications for Therapists and Assistants
Generativity vs. self-absorption or stagnation	Adulthood	Assuming responsible adult roles in community; being worthwhile; looking beyond oneself and embracing future generations	Supportive peers, colleagues, family (including spouse and children), society, community	Important time to include adult in exerting some guiding influence for the next generation; community and social leadership roles
Integrity vs. despair	Older adulthood	Coming to terms with meaning of life; facing mortality and potential despair; feeling satisfaction with one's life	Supportive family (spouse, children, other relatives), friends, religious and community support	Need for a sense of wholeness and vitality; wisdom; respect from others, especially younger people

Adapted from Rainville, E.B. (1999). The special vulnerabilities of children and families. In Poor, S.M. and Rainville, E.B. *Pediatric Therapy: A Systems Approach*. Philadelphia: F.A. Davis Company, with permission.

Life Span Developmental Issues: Implications for Therapists and Assistants: Write in Table

Age Stage	Psychosocial Cognitive Stage	Developmental Task/Key Issues	Important Influences	How can your interaction as a therapist/assistant express sensitivity to these key issues? (Be specific.)
0–2 y	Trust vs. mistrust; Sensorimotor Stage	Attachment; developing trust in self, parents, and world; associating sensory experiences with physical action	Importance of involved caregivers with loving interaction; Importance of some movement experience, repetition and imitation are key.	
2–3 y	Autonomy vs. shame and doubt; beginning of representational thought	Developing feeling of control over behavior; beginning independence and learning of self-control; Understanding symbolism and one-way thought processes	Supportive parents, caregivers, therapists who are supportive, but not threatening; Importance of stimulating language development; imitation and modeling	
2/3 y–6/7 y	Initiative vs. guilt; representational thought	Developing a sense of self and responsibility for one's own actions; initiates own activity	Supportive parents, caregivers , therapists; a time when active exploration should be encouraged; making choices and choosing purposeful activity is vital	

(Continued)

Life Span Developmental Issues: Implications for Therapists and Assistants (*Continued*)

Age Stage	Psychosocial Cognitive Stage	Developmental Task/Key Issues	Important Influences	How can your interaction as a therapist /assistant express sensitivity to these key issues? (Be specific.)
6/7 y–11 y	Industry vs. inferiority; concrete operations	Developing a sense of self-worth through interaction with peers; works on projects for recognition; develops mastery and competence; Ability to solve concrete problems, bound by stimulus and experience	Encouraging educational setting and supportive teachers, caregivers, therapists; need to participate in therapy choices, including goals; value of incentive programs to increase compliance; focus on ability not the disability	
11 y– adolescence	Identity vs. role confusion; formal operations	Developing a strong sense of identity; selecting from among many potential selves; ability to engage in creative problem solving and decision making, including hypothetical thought	Supportive caregivers and teachers, role models and peers; self-esteem and body image are key issues; vocational inquiry	
Young Adulthood	Intimacy vs. isolation	Developing close relationships with others; intimacy and partnership; working toward establishing a career	Supportive peers, colleagues, family (including spouse and children), society; continuing concern regarding self-esteem and sexuality; importance of vocational success	
Adulthood	Generativity vs. self-absorption or stagnation	Assuming responsible adult roles in community; being worthwhile; looking beyond oneself and embracing future generations	Supportive peers, colleagues, family (including spouse and children), society; importance of exerting community and social leadership roles	
Older Adulthood	Integrity vs. despair	Coming to terms with meaning of life; facing mortality and potential despair; feeling satisfaction with one's life	Supportive family (spouse, children, other relatives), friends, religious and community support; need for a sense of wholeness and vitality; wisdom	

Learning Experience Two: Movement Components

Key accomplishments in the developmental acquisition of normal movement components typically include the ability of the body to master antigravity control and strength, the ability to demonstrate proximal stability, and the ability to shift weight effectively to execute a movement or a transitional posture.

■ *Purpose*

In order to "feel" the components of movement, the following exercises can help focus attention on the primary movement components: antigravity control (flexion and extension), proximal stability and weight bearing, weight shifting, rotation, and dissociation.

■ *Materials*

Floor mat or carpeted surface.

■ *Instructions*

Lie on a mat on the floor and close your eyes while the instructor or a colleague verbally guides you through the following movement sequences. As you move, concentrate on your own kinesthetic sense by feeling what muscle groups are firing, the synergists that are being recruited, and when you are literally moving against gravity, stabilizing a body part, shifting your weight, rotating, or dissociating one part of the body from the other. Move at different speeds, and try to gain an appreciation of the fluidity of normal movement and how all of these vital movement components contribute to smooth voluntary movement control.

Example One: Movement in Prone

> Prone on forearms →
> Forearm weight shift to reach →
> Extended arm support →
> Extended arm weight shift to reach →
> Quadruped →
> Weight shifting in quadruped →
> (Side to side, forward and backward, diagonally)
> Reaching from quadruped (weight shift) →
> Upright kneeling →
> Weight shift side to side in kneel →
> Half kneel to both right and left →
> Stand

While moving through this sequence in prone, pay attention to what muscle groups are being activated during the holding portion of each movement (stability) and also during the weight shifts and transitions (mobility). Focus on how the movement components all contribute to normal postural control, upper extremity (UE) control, and lower extremity (LE) control. Concentrate also on the head and trunk control required during these movements and postures.

Example Two: Movement in Supine

> Supine full flexion →
> Transition from supine to side-lying →
> Transition from side-lying or supine to side-sit →
> Transition from side-sit to all fours

While moving through this sequence from supine, pay attention to the amount of flexor antigravity control used and the dissociation and rotation needed for smooth movement. Focus on how the movement components all contribute to normal postural control, UE control, and LE control. Concentrate also on the head and trunk control required during these movements and postures.

Example Three: Functional Activities That Highlight Value of Key Movement Components

Under the guidance of the instructor, practice the following movement activities:

1. Bridging—Used to improve bed mobility, use of bedpan, and assistance with dressing, as well as to aid in the establishment of pelvic control required for LE function, including gait.

2. Weight Shift Activities in Standing—In parallel bars first (then move out of bars), practice weight shift side to side and forward and backward. Concentrate on the contributions of the head and trunk and on the LE control required for this movement.

3. Gait—Demonstrate and practice weight shift to one LE, and then shift forward to opposite LE, advancing; practice stepping forward and backward.

Learning Experience Three: Observation of Movement at Different Life Span Stages

Functional movement is presented in the main text as accomplishments within three broad movement tasks: postural control, UE control and function, and LE control and function. The development of functional movement within these three task areas emerges and changes throughout the life span: infancy and early childhood, middle to late childhood, adolescence, adulthood, and the aging adult. The fundamental movement components of antigravity control, proximal stability, ability to bear weight, smooth weight shift, mobility, and rotation and dissociation can be observed at every life stage as the mover exerts movement control within the environment to carry out age- and task-appropriate skills. Current knowledge indicates that clinicians should consider a patient's age when selecting movement patterns to teach (Ford-Smith and Van Sant, 1993). In addition to age, it is vital to consider body size, body shape, gender, and activity level as all of these variables will affect the selection of the most optimal movement pattern for that person (Van Sant, 1990).

▪ Purpose

If clinicians are sensitive to the developmental phase within which the patient is functioning, effective assessment and intervention strategies can then be designed. The purpose of this exercise is to offer the learner an opportunity to observe movement and how movement changes over the life cycle.

▪ Materials

For this experience, the learners must go out and observe movement in a variety of naturally occurring environmental settings: playgrounds, day care play areas, all levels of schools, swimming programs, amusement parks, yoga classes, shopping malls; the list is endless.

▪ Instructions

In pairs, students are assigned to observe movement of individuals within all of the various age groups. These observations are done from a distance, where the observers are watching the individual engage in an activity without the observed individual knowing. The students record observations about the characteristics of the movement behavior. After all of the observations are completed, the student pair discusses, compares, and contrasts the observable movement behavior of individuals across the life span. The following list offers some suggestions for movement observations, although the students and instructor are invited to use their imagination to add to the list.

Infancy: Infant 8–10-months old playing on the floor, participating in a swimming program, or playing outside in any setting.

Early Childhood Through Late Childhood: Observations from all of these age stages within a similar setting, such as different ages playing on a playground, playing freely in an open outdoor space, or playing in an indoor space, such as a "kid's gym" or recreational setting.

Middle Childhood, Adolescence, and Adults: Observations of all of these individuals playing the same sport, such as baseball or softball; swimming at free play in a pool; playing in the ocean or on the beach.

All ages: Observations of all of these individuals walking in a shopping mall or participating in an exercise class.

The instructor, focusing on the variations and similarities of movement across the life span, then directs analysis and discussion among the members of the entire class.

_____

_____

_____

_____

_____

_____

_____

Learning Experience Four: Automatic Responses

Automatic movements are those that occur in response to a given stimulus, often without conscious, voluntary effort. Automatic movements include reflexes, postural reactions such as righting, equilibrium, protective reactions, and associated reactions. A reflex is a largely automatic, somewhat stereotypical, consistent, and predictable motor response to a specific stimulus, usually sensory (Leonard, 1998). In its broadest sense, a reflex can be defined as a complex motor response pattern, not limited to activation by external stimuli, that, although relatively invariable, is nonetheless responsive to context or environment (Crutchfield and Barnes, 1993; Pimentel, 1996). There is increasing evidence that, rather than being inflexibly paired to a sensory input, if the sensory stimulus is applied during the course of an ongoing movement, the motor output associated with the stimulus will vary, depending on its environmental context and the status of all of the movement subsystems (Field-Fote, 2000). This view is in agreement with a dynamically responsive set of systems contributing to movement.

Consistent with a dynamic systems approach, primitive reflexes are not so much "hardwired" but are readily observed at certain ages; the infant's movement will "under certain circumstances have a propensity [inclination or predisposition] to exhibit a particular motor response" (Kamm et al, 1990). Primitive reflexes always serve some sort of movement purpose. Early in development, they allow for muscle activation, joint excursion, or even provide a primitive survival response. Functionally, primitive reflex responses are thought to contribute to the development of emerging mobility and stability in the developing child.

Automatic movements also include postural responses. Every movement involves a weight shift, and weight shifts in turn, stimulating vestibular and proprioceptive receptors, are the stimulus for righting and equilibrium reactions. Righting and equilibrium are complex postural responses that continue to be present throughout adulthood. Righting behaviors are thought to be mediated at a mid-brain level in response to signaling from several different sensory receptors: proprioceptors and cutaneous receptors, the eyes, and the labyrinths of the ears. Righting is the act of realigning the head or trunk with each other or with regard to an outside stimulus. Applied to movement, righting responses are demonstrated by the head or trunk when balance is disturbed, whereby the head and/or the trunk realign themselves with each other or with respect to the downward pull of gravity. Righting responses assist in keeping the head oriented in relation to the body or to gravity. They are named in a very descriptive fashion, the name telling exactly what body part is responsible for the realignment or righting action and, often, the mechanism for sending this signal. The following are examples of righting responses: head righting, neck righting, and trunk righting. They can be further described by adding a term,

such as labyrinthine head righting or optical head righting (where the stimulus that elicits the righting response is the effect of gravity or the position of the eyes with respect to gravity, respectively).

Equilibrium is the act of reestablishing balance once it is disturbed. Equilibrium reactions adjust for a change in the body's orientation in space. Equilibrium reactions consist of righting responses of the head and trunk and protective extension responses of the extremities. An equilibrium response is composed of head and trunk lateral righting and wide abduction of the UE and LE in the direction away from gravity and a protective extension of the UE and LE toward gravity. The lateral righting and abduction of the head, trunk, and uppermost extremities are the body's attempt to right, realign, or reestablish balance because the center of gravity has moved outside the base of support. The protective extension motions of the lowermost extremities are in preparation for catching oneself from a fall.

Equilibrium reactions develop in increasingly more upright antigravity positions as postural control develops. Therefore, they are seen in the child in prone, supine, sitting, quadruped, kneeling, and finally standing, continuing to mature throughout early childhood as postural control develops (Fisher and Bundy, 1982; Israelevitz et al, 1985). Protective extension also develops as movement control develops, seen as part of an equilibrium response or demonstrated first in sitting with the UEs extending when the infant is displaced forward, to the side, and then to the rear. Functionally, righting and equilibrium reaction responses are thought to contribute to the development of combined mobility and stability in the developing child (McCormack and Perrin, 1997).

Associated reactions are movements that occur involuntarily in accompaniment to another movement. Associated reactions are part of the normal movement repertoire, often observed during a heavily resisted movement or during periods of fatigue or stress. They are common through middle childhood, when postural control and fundamental movement skills are developing and being refined. They are common again whenever the movement system is stressed, such as during recovery from a pathological incident.

▪ Purpose

The purpose of this exercise is to offer the learner an opportunity to demonstrate reflex positions as possible preferred patterns of movement and to experience the demonstration and observation of equilibrium responses.

▪ Materials

Mat table, large gymnastic ball, floor mat or carpeted surface.

▪ Instructions

Reflexes: Using the figures in the text and the following Table 4–2 as your guide, duplicate the position described as a movement response in a reflex pattern, remembering that the demonstration of a reflex pattern may be the preferred pattern of movement seen during a phase of early development or during a period of motor control recovery from a neurological incident.

1. Flexor withdrawal
2. Crossed extension
3. Tonic labyrinthine prone and supine
4. Asymmetrical tonic neck reflex
5. Symmetrical tonic neck reflex
6. Palmar grasp
7. Positive support

TABLE 4–2   Primitive Reflexes

Reflex	Stimulus	Movement Response	Age Typically Observed
Flexor Withdrawal	Stimulus, usually noxious, to sole of foot	Entire LE flexes, ankles dorsiflex, toes extend	28 weeks gestation–1 mo
Crossed Extension	Stimulus, usually noxious, to sole of foot	Opposite LE extends and adducts	28 weeks gestation–1 mo
Rooting	Touch on cheek	Head turn to stimulus, mouth opens	28 weeks gestation–3 mos
Stepping	Upright-supported weight bearing onto firm surface on plantar surface foot	Reciprocal flexion and extension of legs "stepping"	38 weeks gestation–2 mos
Positive Support	Weight onto ball of foot in upright	Stiff extension of LE	35 weeks gestation–2 mos
Moro	Sudden change in head position in relation to trunk	Mass extension and abduction, quickly followed by mass flexion and adduction	28 weeks gestation–6 mos
Startle	Loud, sudden noise	Mass extension and abduction of arms	Birth–persists
Palmar Grasp	Pressure on palm of hand, ulnar side	Strong flexion of fingers	Birth–4 mos
Asymmetrical Tonic Neck Reflex (ATNR)	Rotation of head to one side	Extension of extremities on face side; flexion of extremities on skull side	Birth–6 mos
Symmetrical Tonic Neck Reflex	Flexion or extension of the neck	With neck flexion: flexion of the UEs and extension of the LEs. With neck extension, extension of the UEs and flexion of the LEs	4–12 mos
Tonic Labyrinthine Reflex, supine or prone	Supine or prone position	With supine position: extension of the neck, trunk, and extremities. With prone position: flexion of the neck, trunk, and extremities	Birth–6 mos

Sources: Information compiled from multiple sources. See main text for details and references.

Answer the following questions:

1. How might your recognition of these reflexes, if expressed by your patient/client, influence your approach to this person?

_____

_____

_____

_____

2. How do you think the predominance of these movement patterns may influence functional movement?

_____

_____

_____

_____

Postural responses: Using a gymnastic ball, observe the demonstration of equilibrium reactions in the following positions: prone, supine, sitting. Observe the righting and protective extension responses. Discuss the importance of intact postural response capabilities and how they subserve functional movement control throughout the life span.

_____

_____

_____

_____

Review Questions

1. What is the difference between development, growth, maturation, and adaptation?

2. What is motor development? What is meant by "motor development is a life-span event"?

3. What is the clinical significance of sensitive periods as they occur during development?

4. What is meant by "resiliency" when used to describe the ever-developing individual?

5. Summarize Piaget's theory of cognitive development. How can an understanding of this theory help to make you a more effective clinician?

6. Summarize Erikson's theory of personality development. How can an understanding of this theory help to make you a more effective clinician?

7. Summarize the neuromaturational development theory originated by Gesell. How can an understanding of this theory help to make you a more effective clinician?

_____

_____

_____

_____

8. Summarize the dynamic systems theory's perspective on motor development. How can an understanding of this theory help to make you a more effective clinician?

_____

_____

_____

_____

9. Describe the appropriate use of the following terms related to motor development: cephalocaudal, proximal to distal, gross to fine, undifferentiated to specific. Give an example of each concept applied to motor development.

_____

_____

_____

_____

10. Describe the key concepts embraced by the following kinesiological concepts as related to motor development: physiological flexion to antigravity extension to antigravity flexion, mobility, stability, asymmetry to symmetry to controlled asymmetry, weight bearing, weight shifting, dissociation, rotation. Give an example of each concept applied to motor development.

_____

_____

_____

_____

11. What is the developmental sequence? Why is sequence such a troublesome term to use to describe this process?

_____

_____

_____

_____

12. How does knowledge of motor milestones assist the rehabilitation clinician?

_____

_____

_____

_____

13. Summarize the main gross motor milestones.

14. Summarize the main fine motor milestones.

15. Describe the following types of automatic movements: reflex, righting reaction, equilibrium reaction, protective extension, associated reactions. Give an example of each.

16. What is meant by "functional movement"?

17. Describe the main functional movement components required for successful postural control of the head and trunk.

18. Describe the main functional movement components required for successful UE control.

19. Describe the main functional movement components required for successful LE control.

20. Using the first year of life as a model, describe the development of postural control, UE control and manipulation, and LE control and locomotion. Highlight key changes over the first year, focusing on the process of development.

_____

_____

_____

_____

21. Describe the major developmental changes in the development of postural control, UE control, and LE control that occur during early childhood, middle to late childhood, adolescence, and adulthood.

_____

_____

_____

_____

22. Describe the major developmental changes during aging in postural control, UE control, and LE control.

_____

_____

_____

_____

Motor Learning Through the Life Span

Effective therapists think of themselves as teachers or facilitators of human movement education or reeducation. Patients are learners and are, therefore, students. It is imperative that physical and occupational therapists and assistants use effective teaching and learning strategies when working with patients/clients. Motor learning is a process that brings about a relatively permanent change in the capacity for motor performance. Three major factors that affect motor learning are environmental conditions, cognitive processes, and movement organization (Jarus, 1994) Occupational and physical therapy intervention involves all the fundamental characteristics of motor learning: clinicians provide instruction, feedback, opportunities to practice, and encouragement to patients. Therapists and assistants use teaching strategies such as instruction, practice, and feedback to guide patients through skill mastery. An understanding of motor learning will enhance the clinician's ability to view the patient/client as the learner and therefore enable the clinician to be most effective in maximizing functional rehabilitation for that person. Patients will achieve maximal progress when therapy is guided by principles of motor learning.

Active Learning Experiences

Learning Experience One: Learning a Novel Motor Skill

When teaching a motor skill, several factors are to be considered when structuring the learning activity. These key elements are the environment; the level of arousal, attention, and motivation of the learner; and the use of instruction, guidance, practice, and feedback. A gifted teacher (clinician) can effectively modify and manipulate these variables to create the most optimal learning opportunity for the patient.

▪ Purpose

This exercise explores the ways a learning experience is structured for a novel task or the refinement and practice of a familiar or previously learned task. Different strategies are used by the teacher and the learner depending on the task itself and the stage of learning.

▪ Materials

None.

▪ Instructions

The instructor or your partner teaches you a new dance step. As the teacher guides you through skill mastery, note how the learning experience is structured (or actually unstructured at the later stages of learning). How does the teacher use and set up the following elements of the learning situation:

- Environment

_____

_____

_____

_____

- Instruction and guidance

_____

_____

_____

_____

- Practice: physical or mental, part or whole, constant or varied

_____

_____

_____

_____

- Feedback: how often, how much, and when; what type.

_____

_____

_____

_____

The teacher then sends you home to practice; upon return at a later time, the learning experience for that same skill is structured differently, now that perhaps you have developed some level of skill mastery. The teacher will proceed with this active learning experience until you are extremely skilled. How has the instructor effectively used teaching strategies to facilitate your learning of this motor skill?

_____

_____

_____

Repeat this entire process, now with you as the instructor, teaching a novel motor skill to a friend. Expand this activity by repeating this experience and teaching a similar skill to a toddler, a young adolescent, an adult, and an older adult. Compare and contrast how teaching and learning strategies are individualized for different persons.

_____

_____

_____

_____

This learning experience can be expanded and explored with countless variations. Have fun!

Learning Experience Two: Stages of Learning

As depicted in Table 5–3 in the main text, there are differences between conditions that promote skill acquisition (initial learning) and those that promote retention and transfer (long-term learning). The skilled clinician (motor learning teacher) is adept at recognizing where the patient (learner) is along the continuum of learning and effectively modifies conditions appropriately.

▪ Purpose

The purpose of this learning experience is to practice the application and modification of setting up the environment, using practice, guidance, and feedback for different learners at different ages and different stages of learning, with learners who are compromised by a damaged neurological system.

▪ Materials

Wheelchair, quad cane, stairs with railing.

▪ Instructions

For the following three patients, discuss and demonstrate how you would set up the most optimal motor learning experience for that patient at that phase of learning and at that age stage. Engage in this activity by role-playing in small groups, where one person is the patient and the others are the therapist and assistant. Keep in mind the cognitive, sensory, and musculoskeletal impairments that also contribute to this patient's individual clinical picture. The emphasis of this learning experience is on your teaching strategies as a clinician, but this same experience can be used to practice actual intervention techniques, if you have mastery of some of those skills. Because the intent of this learning experience is to emphasize teaching and learning strategies for different learning stages, the author is purposely describing three patients who present with a hemiplegia, without introducing the variable of different pathological conditions and impairments, and how that specific condition may affect learning. The author has also described three adults, but changing the ages of the imagined patients and introducing the variable of learners of different ages can expand this learning experience.

Primarily, you are asked to focus on the use of learning strategies. The author recognizes that it is within the practice scope of the _therapist_ to set goals and design interventions; the role of the _assistant_ is to participate in this decision making and carry out the intervention within the established plan of care. The learning experience described herein is considered to be of value for _both_ levels of professional because of the close working relationship and the importance of teamwork within the practice setting.

TABLE 5–1	**Learning Styles**	
Learning Style	Characteristics	Strengths of Style
Diverging	"People with this learning style are best at viewing concrete situations from many different points of view. Their approach to situations is to observe rather than take action. If this is your style, you enjoy brainstorming sessions. You probably have broad cultural interests, are imaginative, sensitive to feelings, and like to gather information. In formal learning situations, you prefer working in groups, listening with an open mind, and receiving personalized feedback."	Being imaginative Understanding people Recognizing problems Brainstorming Being open-minded
Assimilating	" People with this learning style are best at understanding a wide range of information and putting it into concise, logical form. If this is your learning style, you are probably less focused on people and more interested in ideas and concepts. People with this style of learning find it more important that a theory have logical soundness than practical value. This style is important for effectiveness in information and science careers. In formal learning situations, you may prefer formal lectures, readings, and having time to think things through."	Planning Creating models Defining problems Developing theories Being patient
Converging	"People with this learning style are best at finding practical uses for ideas and theories. If this is your preferred learning style, you have the ability to solve problems and make decisions based on finding solutions to questions or problems. You would rather deal with technical tasks ands problems than with social and interpersonal issues. These skills are important for effectiveness in specialist and technology careers. In formal learning situations, you prefer to experiment with new ideas, laboratory assignments, and practical applications."	Solving problems Making decisions Reasoning deductively Defining problems Being logical
Accommodating	"People with this learning style have the ability to learn primarily from hands-on experience. If this is your style, you probably enjoy carrying out plans and involving yourself in new and challenging experiences. You may tend to react on "gut" feelings rather than on a logical analysis. In solving problems, you rely more heavily on people for information than on your own technical analysis. This style is important for effectiveness in action-oriented careers such as marketing or sales. In formal learning situations, you prefer to work with others to get assignments done, to set goals, to do field work, or to test out different approaches for completing a project" (Kolb, 1999).	Getting things done Leading Taking risks Initiating Being adaptable and practical

Excerpted from Kolb,1999, with permission from the Hay Group.

Case Example One

Mrs. A is a 75-year-old woman recently admitted to the hospital with a left hemiplegia secondary to a right CVA, sustained last week. She lives at home with her spouse of 53 years and is a retired music teacher. She is confused but pleasant. Mrs. A presents to you seated in a wheelchair, leaning completely off midline with apparent trunk control limitations, seeming to ignore her left side.

> Muscle Tone/Strength: Muscle tone and strength of right side is within functional limits. The left upper extremity is flaccid, with an obvious shoulder subluxation. The left lower extremity presents with emerging spasticity; the only voluntary movements able to be demonstrated by Mrs. A are the initiation of abduction and flexion at hip, partial knee extension and ankle plantar flexion, especially when supported in the upright position.

> ROM: Subluxation of the left shoulder, all upper extremity range within normal limits; left ankle dorsiflexion just to neutral with knee extended.

> Function: Supported and unsupported balance in sitting is poor; absence of protective responses left upper extremity; apparently limited integration of both body sides into body scheme.

Questions for Case Example One

For this clinical scenario, the following questions can be answered to help guide discussion.

1. Chose a main functional goal for this imaginary patient. What functional task will you concentrate on, and how will you go about retraining for that task for this patient at this phase of rehabilitation? Different student groups could choose a different goal for the same patient, or the instructor could choose one for the entire class.

_____

_____

_____

2. Conjure up a mental image of this patient. In what phase of learning do you picture this individual generally presenting?

_____

_____

_____

3. What is the best learning environment for this patient? Describe in detail, and simulate.

_____

_____

_____

4. What forms of learning (nonassociative and associative) do you intend to try to establish with this patient? Describe some clinical strategies or methods that might help activate this type of learning process.

_____

_____

_____

5. How will you use or not use instruction and guidance?

_____

_____

_____

6. Feedback: what type of feedback will you give and how?

_____

_____

_____

7. Practice: what practice conditions are most appropriate for this patient?

_____

_____

_____

Case Example Two

Mr. B is a 55-year-old man undergoing rehabilitation for a left hemiplegia secondary to a right cerebrovascular accident 3 weeks ago. He has just retired from a nearby college, where he was a psychology professor for 30 years. He lives alone with several pets and has spent most of his time in recent years writing and publishing his work. He presents to you with a flat affect and appears to be very depressed. Mr. B arrives in this rehabilitation center in a wheelchair, which he self-propels.

Muscle Tone/Strength: Muscle tone is characterized by hypertonicity throughout both left extremities, with predominant flexor tone in the upper extremity and extensor tone in the lower extremity. He has just begun to demonstrate some voluntary movements in the left extremities, although these isolated attempts are inconsistent. Strength on the right side is with functional limits; in fact, Mr. B was an outdoorsman and was very active physically before his stroke.

ROM: There are minimal limitations in range of motion as follows: left shoulder: flexion 0° to 115° and abduction 0° to 65°. Shoulder motion is accompanied by pain.

Function: Supported sitting is stable. Mr. B uses his left body side when reminded but not automatically. He stands with maximal assist of one person and is still working on preambulation tasks.

Questions for Case Example Two

For each of these clinical scenarios, the following questions can be answered to help guide discussion.

1. Choose a main functional goal for this imaginary patient. What functional task will you concentrate on, and how will you go about retraining for that task for this patient at this phase of rehabilitation? Different student groups could choose a different goal for the same patient, or the instructor could choose one for the entire class.

_____

_____

_____

2. Conjure up a mental image of this patient. In what phase of learning do you picture this individual generally presenting?

_____

_____

_____

3. What is the best learning environment for this learner? Describe in detail, and simulate.

_____

_____

_____

4. What forms of learning (nonassociative and associative) do you intend to try to establish with this patient? Describe some clinical strategies or methods that might help activate that type of learning process.

_____

_____

_____

5. How will you use or not use instruction and guidance?

_____

_____

6. Feedback: what type of feedback will you give and how?

_____

_____

_____

7. Practice: what practice conditions are most appropriate for this patient?

_____

_____

_____

Case Example Three

Mrs. C is a 72-year-old woman attending outpatient therapy for a left hemiplegia secondary to a right cerebrovascular accident suffered 3 months ago. She lives in a one-story home with two steps front access with her daughter and three grandsons. She was an interior decorator and continues to enjoy crafts. Mrs. C is alert and oriented but is beginning to show signs of senile dementia.

Muscle Tone/Strength: Mrs. C has voluntary, isolated movements on the left side, but generally strength function is just at a grade of three, antigravity capability. Movement patterns are characterized by residual evidence of spasticity and associated reactions in both left extremities, accompanying stress and effort.

ROM: Range of motion on the right is within functional limits. Limitations in range of motion are present in both left extremities as follows: shoulder flexion 20° to 145° with pain; wrist extension to neutral only.

Function: Mrs. C ambulates with close supervision and is demonstrating several persisting gait deviations, using a quad cane. She requires moderate assistance on stairs mostly because she is extremely anxious when presented with stairs.

Questions for Case Example Three

For this clinical scenario, the following questions can be answered to help guide discussion.

1. Choose a main functional goal for this imaginary patient. What functional task will you concentrate on, and how will you go about retraining for that task for this patient at this phase of rehabilitation? Different student groups could choose a different goal for the same patient, or the instructor could choose one for the entire class.

   _____

   _____

   _____

2. Conjure up a mental image of this patient. In what phase of learning do you picture this individual generally presenting?

   _____

   _____

   _____

3. What is the best learning environment for this learner? Describe in detail and simulate.

   _____

   _____

   _____

4. What forms of learning (nonassociative and associative) do you intend to try to establish with this patient? Describe some clinical strategies or methods that might help activate that type of learning process?

   _____

   _____

   _____

5. How will you use or not use instruction and guidance?

   _____

   _____

   _____

6. Feedback: what type of feedback will you give and how?

   _____

   _____

   _____

7. Practice: what practice conditions are most appropriate for this patient?

   _____

   _____

   _____

Learning Experience Three: What is Your Learning Style?

The following are the main tenets applicable to teaching the adult learner in physical and occupational therapy:

- An adult's readiness to learn depends on his or her previous learning.
- Intrinsic motivation produces more pervasive and permanent learning.
- Positive reinforcement is highly effective and preferred by adult learners.
- Material to be learned needs to be presented in an organized fashion.
- Learning is enhanced by repetition.
- Tasks that are more meaningful are more fully and easily learned.
- Active participation in learning improves retention.
- Environmental factors affect learning.
- Adults exhibit learning styles that illustrate various learning theories, such as :
  1. Having personal strategies for coding information. ("I need to process and remember this *my* way.")
  2. Perceiving in different ways.
  3. Perceiving learning activities as problem-centered and relevant to life.
  4. Desiring some immediate appreciation.
  5. Having a concept of themselves as learners.
  6. Being self-directed.

Therapists and assistants are encouraged to engage in a dialogue with an adult learner to discover that individual adult's unique learning style. Learning style refers to how information is processed by and is unique to an individual (Kolb, 1999; Dunn et al, 1981). Readers are encouraged to learn more about learning styles and how an individual's style will influence learning in the therapeutic environment. Therapeutic interaction that attempts to complement that learning style will be more effective (Avers and Gardner, 2000). Kolb's Learning Style Inventory (1999) describes four different types of learning styles, which are outlined in Table 5–1.

▪ *Purpose*

The purpose of this exercise is to offer the learner an opportunity to explore the concept of learning styles, including one's own. Discussions about the clinical implication are of prime importance.

▪ *Materials*

None.

▪ *Instructions*

Read the descriptions of learning styles in Table 5–1, and try to discern what your learning style is as an adult learner. As a potential patient in a physical therapy or occupational therapy clinic, how would you like to be taught? Discuss clinical implications as a group. Discuss these concepts with a partner. As prompted by these concepts, explain to your partner, in your own words, how you think you learn.

DISCUSSION: _____

_____

_____

_____

_____

_____

Learning Experience Four: Case Studies Revisited

Review the case studies presented at the end of the chapter in the textbook. With a partner, role-play the teaching and learning interaction as it is described. Critique the case study, and discuss as a group how you as the clinician would use the elements of learning (environmental setting, instructions and guidance, practice, and feedback) differently than described in the case study. Recognize the value of individualizing teaching strategies and how you, as the teacher (therapist), might help the learner (patient) progress differently through the described learning process.

Case Study: Child: _____

_____

_____

_____

_____

_____

_____

_____

_____

_____

_____

_____

Case Study: Adult: _____

_____

_____

_____

_____

_____

_____

_____

_____

_____

_____

_____

_____

_____

_____

Review Questions

1. What is learning? What are the differences between learning, training, and performance?

2. What is the difference between motor control and motor learning? What are the unique contributions that each area of knowledge makes to intervention with patients with impaired movement?

3. What are the basic cellular processes that are involved in learning and the establishment of long-term memory?

4. Describe the following different types of nonassociative learning, giving a clinical example of each: habituation, sensitization, perceptual learning.

5. Describe the following different types of associative learning, giving a clinical example of each: classical conditioning, operant conditioning, procedural learning, declarative learning.

6. What are the salient concepts from the following motor learning theories: Adam's Closed-Loop theory, Schmidt's Schema Theory, Ecological Theory?

7. Describe some of the key concepts to be considered in setting up the most appropriate therapeutic environment for patient/client learning?

_____

_____

_____

_____

8. What is meant by arousal, attention, and motivation, and what is the effect of each of these factors on patient/client learning?

_____

_____

_____

_____

9. How can a clinician effectively use instruction and guidance in teaching a patient/client a movement skill?

_____

_____

_____

_____

10. What is feedback and what are the different types of feedback? What kind of factors should a clinician consider in the selection and timing of feedback for a patient?

_____

_____

_____

_____

11. Define practice, the different types of practice, and the clinical considerations to be given to the organization of practice.

_____

_____

_____

_____

12. What are some of the main characteristics of a patient who is in the cognitive stage of learning? How can a clinician enhance patient learning in this stage?

_____

_____

_____

_____

13. What are some of the main characteristics of a patient who is in the associative stage of learning? How can a clinician enhance patient learning in this stage?

_____

_____

_____

_____

14. What are some of the main characteristics of a patient who is in the autonomous stage of learning? How can a clinician enhance patient learning in this stage?

_____

_____

_____

_____

15. How can a clinician apply the key concepts presented by Gentile (1992), presented as the two stages of learning? What is meant by the following terms: open versus closed skills, regulatory and nonregulatory conditions, explicit and implicit learning?

_____

_____

_____

_____

16. What is the value of learning in a natural environment? Why is it thought that learning is enhanced when the learner understands the importance of tasks with added-purpose, occupational embeddedness, and goal-directed activity? Highlight how this knowledge can affect therapeutic intervention and effective structuring of a therapy session.

_____

_____

_____

_____

17. What are some of the main characteristics that are relevant to the child as a learner? What are the implications for therapeutic teaching strategies?

_____

_____

_____

_____

18. What are some of the main characteristics that are relevant to the adult as a learner? What are the implications for therapeutic teaching strategies?

_____

_____

_____

_____

19. What are some of the key issues regarding learning opportunities and challenges of the older adult? What are the implications for therapeutic teaching strategies?

_____

_____

_____

_____

20. How can a clinician maximize an optimal learning opportunity for individuals with cognitive impairment, including children with mental retardation?

_____

_____

_____

_____

21. Summarize important learning issues to be considered in the teaching of individuals presenting with the common pathological conditions of brain injury, post-cerebrovascular accident, or Parkinson's disease.

_____

_____

_____

_____

Neurorehabilitation Intervention Approaches

6

Therapeutic approaches to intervention with individuals with neurological disorders have evolved over the past several decades since the creation of the professions of occupational and physical therapy. These patient-centered rehabilitation professions of physical therapy and occupational therapy are dynamic, constantly building on an ever-growing body of neuroscience knowledge. Approaches to patient intervention or frames of reference naturally emerge and develop as the base of knowledge broadens. It is crucial that the treating clinician (therapist or therapist assistant) develop an ability to make sound clinical decisions in selecting from among these sometimes diverse approaches and interventions in order to offer the patient the best approach possible. Furthermore, it is reasonable to expect that therapeutic approaches to intervention will *continue* to emerge, develop, and become refined. Critical thinking is a *must* for the contemporary clinician, who is charged with staying abreast of new knowledge and, therefore, innovative intervention opportunities.

Treatment or intervention approaches emerge as a result of the interface between theory and clinical problem solving. Therapists and assistants are encouraged to study the contributions from each approach and become eclectic in an approach to patient care. It is rarely best for the patient that a clinician be proficient in only one intervention approach. Although current scientific knowledge undoubtedly encourages therapists to prioritize a dynamic systems approach and the importance of functional movement, new knowledge will continue to emerge. Therefore, *any* current theory of motor control with an accompanying clinical intervention model is in a sense unfinished, because there must always be room to revise and incorporate new information, knowledge, and insights.

No one approach offers all of the answers or is the best choice for all patients/clients of any age who present with the plethora of clinical dilemmas encountered. Although many of the original tenets of some earlier intervention approaches have now been abandoned, there is value in some of their insights.

Clinicians are responsible for assimilating key patient information and choosing relevant concepts from varying frames of reference to solve commonly encountered clinical problems. The most effective clinicians are problem solving, informed, and eclectic, constantly searching for the closest match between the presenting patient's main movement problem and the tools that are available to help the patient optimize functional performance, independence, and well-being. The best approach to a patient is most often an integrated one, assimilating all types of information, and deriving an individual, patient-centered custom approach. The choice of interventions must be function-based and have the greatest chance of promoting successful motor function for the unique individual person.

Both the occupational therapy and physical therapy professions have a Guide to practice, offering practitioners a concrete method for moving through the clinical decision making necessary to most efficiently optimize a *functional outcome* for the patient. Most physical and occupational therapists currently subscribe to an eclectic approach to intervention, selecting aspects from several different approaches or frames of reference in order to meet the individual needs of the patient. The main emphasis in both physical and occupational therapy is on a functional approach to assessment and intervention.

Active Learning Experiences

Learning Experience One: Integrated Use of Sensorimotor "Hands-On" Techniques

The manual techniques that originally developed as a result of the early reflex and hierarchical theories can be useful as incorporated into a total treatment or intervention approach. Readers are requested to consult the text for current concepts regarding these intervention approaches.

▪ *Purpose*

This exercise offers the learner an opportunity to practice techniques and to role-play incorporating these manual techniques into patient treatment or intervention.

▪ *Materials*

None.

▪ *Instructions*

Proprioceptive neuromuscular facilitation (PNF): Using Table 6–1, practice performing the PNF diagonals as demonstrated by the course instructor or demonstrated originally in Knott and Voss (1968) or in a current therapeutic exercise textbook. The following suggestions are offered to guide your mastery of manual contacts.

TABLE 6–1	**Summary of Stimulation Techniques Used During PNF and Application to Intervention**	
Stimulation Technique	Application	Goal and Presumed Benefit
Manual Contacts	Pressure is given to the skin over the muscle being facilitated.	Manually contacting the patient utilizes sensory cues to direct the patient's attention to the desired movement. Pressure activates mechanoreceptors.
Vision	Patient is asked to watch the movement and to participate in giving the movement direction.	Visually directed movement is used as reinforcement and to offer extrinsic feedback to the patient as he or she learns the movement.
Verbal Commands	Tone of voice and specific commands are used selectively to prepare the patient for movement, to direct the movement, and to motivate the patient.	Voice is used to affect the quality of the patient's response. Tone and timing of commands are used as teaching aids.
Stretch	Quick stretch is given to the muscle being facilitated. Stretch can be applied at the beginning of the motion or intermittently throughout the range of motion to activate or reinforce muscle activation/contraction.	Quick stretch activates the muscle spindle and excites the agonist muscle through activation of the monosynaptic reflex arc.
Traction	Separation of the joint surfaces to activate joint receptors.	A traction stimulus activates proprioceptive joint receptors, theorized to promote movement.
Approximation	Compression of joint surfaces, usually done with the body part in a weight-bearing position.	Used to activate proprioceptive joint receptors to promote muscular co-contraction, joint stability, and weight bearing.
Resistance	Resistance given to an active contraction; resistance can be graded or maximal, depending on the movement goal.	Used to increase muscular strength, reinforce a contraction, or to induce irradiation (spread) of the contraction to synergists.
Timing	Timing is selectively used by the therapist to either facilitate motor learning as the patient recognizes the familiarity of a frequently used movement pattern (normal timing) or to emphasize a specific portion of the movement pattern (timing for emphasis).	The movement patterns used in PNF are based on typically occurring patterns of normal movement used in work and sports. Timing is an important component of learning a movement pattern.
Rhythmic Stabilization	Rhythmic, alternating isometric contractions of agonist and antagonist without intermittent relaxation; resistance is carefully graded to achieve co-contraction.	Used to promote weight bearing and holding and to improve postural stability, strength, and proximal control.

Sources: Information compiled from multiple sources. See main text for details and references.

▪ Suggestions for Learning Manual Contacts

Practice placing hands on your partner for a specific pattern. Have partner move actively through the available range of motion. Using your hands on your partner, manually guide through the diagonal. The following questions are intended for discussion between the learner partners or to assist the learner in assessing his or her own performance.

- Did the positions of your hands allow the full range of motion to occur or did they impede the range of motion?
- Did you move as the subject moved? Was your body in line with the diagonal direction of the movement?
- Were your hands accurately placed so that the pressure was over the muscle groups, tendons, and joints participating in the movement?

Practice using some of the stimulation techniques described in Table 6–1: quick stretch, traction, approximation, resistance, timing, rhythmic stabilization. When are these techniques clinically helpful and appropriate? When are they inappropriate and perhaps counterproductive?

_____

_____

_____

_____

▪ Commands and Communication

- Did my hands and my words help my partner understand what was expected?
- Did I rely too much on too many words rather than on careful use of my hands?
- Did I command my partner to "push" or "pull" when I meant the opposite or I actually meant for him or her to hold?
- Did my partner perform in accordance with normal timing?
- Did my commands encourage normal timing?
- Were my commands directed at the point of emphasis in the diagonal?
- Would the partner's response have been better if I had used a stronger tone of voice?
- Did I use vision as a helpful learning tool?

▪ Manual Facilitation and Inhibition Techniques

Using Tables 6–2 and 6–3 as guides, practice using manual facilitation and inhibition techniques to elicit a response from your partner. Use these sensorimotor techniques within a functional position. Practice including sensorimotor manual techniques into the teaching of a functional movement or encouraging an active response from the patient. Role-play the following clinical examples to illustrate the application of manual techniques in a treatment or intervention plan.

TABLE 6–2	**Treatment Application of Developmental Sequence Concepts**
Position	Treatment Benefits
Supine	• Facilitation of head and upper trunk forward flexion • Can begin early weight-bearing, knees bent, feet flat on surface • For children, can foster visual and upper extremity development
Side lying	• Neutral position of head and neck decreases effect of tonic reflexes, if problematic • Promotes protraction of scapula and hip, important for functional use in upper and lower extremities • Achieves trunk elongation on weight-bearing side • Excellent position to promote rolling, coming to sit, or as transitional posture
Prone on elbows or forearms	• Improves upper trunk, neck and head control • Promotes weight-bearing through upper extremities • Increases co-contraction and proximal stability at shoulder girdle • Increases range of motion at hip and knee extensors

(Continued)

TABLE 6–2	**Treatment Application of Developmental Sequence Concepts** (*Continued*)
Position	Treatment Benefits
Quadruped	• Improves upper and lower trunk, upper and lower extremity, and head/neck control • Improves co-contraction strength of abdominals and back extensors. Trunk works against gravity • Increases hip stabilizer strength • Weight bearing to increase proximal stability at shoulder girdles and hips • Weight bearing through extended arms • Increases extensor range at wrists and fingers • Wide base of support, lowered center of gravity • Excellent opportunity for dissociation and reciprocal extremity movements
Sitting	• Promotes active head and trunk control, trunk elongation and rotation • Excellent for facilitating head and trunk righting, equilibrium responses, upper extremity protective reactions
Side sit with forearm or extended arm prop	• Increases upper extremity strength on weight-bearing side • Improves trunk rotation and dissociation • Offers opportunity for balanced sitting with narrowed base of support
Bridging in supine	• Improves lower trunk and lower extremity control • Increases hip stabilizer strength • Weight bearing through feet • Functional activity to assist with bed mobility
Kneeling and half kneeling	• Improves head/neck, upper and lower trunk, and lower extremity control • Weight bearing through hips • Increases hip stabilizer strength and control • Improves balance reactions • Weight bearing through foot in half kneel • Narrow base of support, higher center of gravity • Encourages dissociation, good transitional postures
Standing	• Improves head/neck, trunk, and lower extremity control • Weight bearing through lower extremities • Improves balance reactions • Narrow base of support, high center of gravity • Functional posture

Excerpted and adapted, with permission, from O'Sullivan, S.B. (2001). Assessment of Motor Function. In O'Sullivan, S.B. & Schmitz, TJ (Eds.). Physical Rehabilitation: Assessment and Treatment, 4th ed. Philadelphia: F. A. Davis Company; and Martin S. and Kessler, M.K. (2000), with permission from Elsevier.

TABLE 6–3	**Manual Facilitation and Inhibition Techniques**			
Technique	Receptor	Stimulus	Response	Comments
Quick Stretch	Muscle spindle Ia endings detect length and velocity changes	Quick stretch or tapping over a muscle belly or tendon	Activates agonist to contract; reciprocal innervation effect will inhibit the antagonist; activates synergists	Response is temporary; can add resistance to augment response; not appropriate to use in muscles where increased muscle tone limits function
Prolonged Stretch	Muscle spindle Ia and II endings; Golgi tendon organs	Maintained stretch in a lengthened range	Muscle contraction dampened (inhibited)	Rationale for serial casting and splinting; to increase the effect; activate the antagonist

TABLE 6–3   Manual Facilitation and Inhibition Techniques

Technique	Receptor	Stimulus	Response	Comments
Resistance	Muscle spindles	Resistance given manually or with body weight or gravity; mechanical weights	Enhances muscle contraction through recruitment; facilitates synergists; enhances kinesthetic awareness	Resistance needs to be graded depending on patient response and goal; additional recruitment and overflow may be counterproductive to movement goal
Approximation	Joint receptors	Compression of joint surfaces: manual or mechanical; bouncing; applied in weight bearing	Enhances muscular co-contraction, proximal stability, and postural extension; increases kinesthetic awareness and postural stability	Effective in combination with rhythmic stabilization (see PNF); contraindicated in inflamed joints
Traction	Joint receptors	Joint surfaces distracted, usually manually and at the beginning of a movement	Facilitates muscle activation to improve mobility and movement initiation	Useful to activate initial mobility. Also used by qualified practitioners as part of mobilization
Inhibitory Pressure	Golgi tendon organs, muscle spindles, tactile receptors	Firm pressure manually or with body weight over muscle belly or tendon	Inhibits muscle activity; dampening effect	Equipment can be used to achieve effect: casts and splints, placing cones in hands; positional use of wheelchair lap tray; weight-bearing activities can provide inhibitory pressure: for example, onto open hand to inhibit finger flexors
Light Touch	Rapidly adapting tactile receptors, autonomic nervous system (sympathetic division)	Brief, light contact to skin	Increased arousal, withdrawal response	Effective in initiating a generalized movement response; to elicit arousal; contraindicated with agitated patients or where autonomic nervous system is unstable
Maintained Touch	Slowly adapting tactile receptors, autonomic nervous system (parasympathetic division)	Maintained contact or pressure	Calming effect, desensitizes skin, general inhibition	Useful for patients with high level of arousal or hypersensitivity
Manual Contacts	Tactile receptors, muscle proprioceptors	Firm, deep pressure of hands over body area	Facilitates contraction of muscle underneath hands	Activates muscle response; enhances sensory and kinesthetic awareness; provides security and support

(Continued)

TABLE 6–3	**Manual Facilitation and Inhibition Techniques** (*Continued*)			
Technique	Receptor	Stimulus	Response	Comments
Slow Stroking	Tactile receptors, autonomic nervous system (parasympathetic division)	Slow, firm stroking with a flat hand over neck or trunk extensors	Calming effect; general inhibition; induces feeling of security	Appropriate for overly aroused patients
Neutral Warmth	Thermoreceptors, autonomic nervous system (parasympathetic division)	Towel or Ace wrap of body or body parts (warm)	General relaxation and inhibition; decreased muscle tone; decreased agitation or pain	Use for 10–15 minutes; avoid overheating. Appropriate for highly agitated patients or individuals with increased sympathetic response
Slow vestibular stimulation	Tonic vestibular receptors	Slow rocking, slow movement on ball, in hammock, in rocking chair	Calming effect; decreased arousal; generalized inhibition	Useful for patients who are defensive to sensory stimulation, hyperreactive to stimulation, hypertonic, or agitated
Fast vestibular stimulation	Semicircular canals	Fast or irregular movement with an acceleration and deceleration component, such as spinning, use of a scooter board, fast rolling	Facilitates general muscle tone and promotes postural responses to movement	Used with patients with hypotonia (cerebral palsy, Down syndrome); used to promote sensory integration (requires specialized training and certification)

Excerpted with permission from O'Sullivan, 2001.

1. Patient displays hypotonia throughout head/ neck, trunk, and extremities. With patient/ client prone on elbows, use stroking and tapping on upper back and neck paraspinal extensors to facilitate neck extension. Remember to use a functional goal to encourage patient interest and motivation.

   _____

   _____

   _____

   _____

2. Patient presents with a right hemiplegia secondary to a left cardiovascular accident, displaying spasticity throughout the right upper extremity. Generally, this patient is clinically presenting as described in stage 3 of recovery (Martin and Kessler, 2000; McKeough, 1999). The right upper extremity is postured into a flexion synergy (Table 6–4) so strong that the therapist or assistant is having difficulty assisting the patient to extend the right arm down onto the wheelchair armrest so that beginning transfer training can occur. Use inhibitory pressure to the biceps to inhibit spasticity in conjunction with gently tapping onto the triceps to encourage elbow extension. Combine this with stroking to facilitate wrist and finger extension and approximation around the shoulder girdle to encourage co-contraction and proximal stability.

   _____

   _____

   _____

   _____

3. Patient has sustained a fall and is presenting with a paraparesis (weakness in both lower extremities). Patient displays weakness of both hip flexors and hip extensors (manual muscle test grade :P or 2). Use quick stretch to initiate and sustain hip flexion and hip extension

TABLE 6–4	**Common Synergy Patterns in Patients Following Stroke**	
Synergy	Description	Significance in Clinical Presentation
Upper Extremity Flexion	Scapula retraction and/or elevation, shoulder external rotation, shoulder abduction (90°), elbow flexion, forearm supination, wrist and finger flexion	Most prevalent synergy pattern seen in the upper extremity; strongest components are scapula retraction and elbow flexion
Upper Extremity Extension	Scapula protraction, shoulder internal rotation, shoulder adduction, elbow extension, forearm pronation, wrist and finger flexion	Not as common a pattern in the upper extremity; shoulder internal rotation and adduction, forearm pronation most common components
Lower Extremity Flexion	Hip flexion, abduction, and external rotation; knee flexion, ankle dorsiflexion with inversion, toe extension	Prevalent pattern when the patient is in a nonweight-bearing position; strongest component is hip flexion
Lower Extremity Extension	Hip extension, adduction, and internal rotation; knee extension, ankle plantarflexion with inversion, toe flexion	Prevalent pattern when the patient is in upright or weight-bearing position; strongest components are knee extension and plantar flexion with inversion

Sources: Data from Brunnstrom, S. (1970). Movement therapy in hemiplegia: A neurophysiological approach. New York: Harper & Row; Martin, S., & Kessler, M. (2000). Neurological intervention for physical therapist assistants. Philadelphia: W. B. Saunders; S. B. O' Sullivan & T. J. Schmitz (Eds.). (2000). Physical rehabilitation: Assessment and treatment (4th ed.). Philadelphia: F. A. Davis; and Sawner, K., & LaVigne, J. (1992). Brunnstrom's movement therapy in hemiplegia (2nd ed.). NewYork: J. B. Lippincott.

throughout the available range of motion. Incorporate tapping to the targeted muscle bellies to reinforce the movement. What functional position would you use for increasing active hip flexion; for active hip extension?

_____

_____

_____

▪ *Neurodevelopmental Treatment (NDT)*

Using Table 6–5 as a guide, practice using manual guidance (handling) and key points of control to facilitate and encourage functional movements, especially transitional movements during active, guided movement. Demonstrate the transitions described in Learning Experience Two in Chapter Four (page 45 this workbook), using your hands and verbal cues as needed. Encourage and observe practice of the transition taught. At times, it may be best to use the partner's shoulder or the pelvis as a key point of control. Try both and experiment. Observation of your partner's responses is most important. Experiment with facilitating weight shift and rotation/dissociation during the movement. Afterwards, ask your partner what your manual guidance felt like. What is encouraging to movement

or counterproductive? Did your guidance help the mover to feel secure to use his or her own available active movements?

Learning Experience Two: Task Analysis and Functional Goals

A contemporary frame of reference for intervention is described in a task-oriented model or treatment approach. Because movement is normally goal-directed, functional tasks are thought to be a natural way to achieve or promote motor control. The task-oriented model is based on the idea that the movement system must solve problems to accomplish motor tasks (Horak, 1991). This model assumes that movement control is organized around goal-directed functional behaviors rather than specific muscles or movement patterns. Recognizing that tasks can be accomplished in more than one way, individuals are encouraged to actively problem-solve and to learn alternative movement patterns that can then be used in a variety of environments. The clinician's role is to provide feedback while manipulating environmental and musculoskeletal demands to help promote the emergence of smooth and efficient functional behaviors (Horak, 1991; Poole, 1997). Movement execution can be accomplished or modified by controlling the degrees of freedom, sometimes as offered by the underlying impairment (limited range

TABLE 6–5	**Summary of NDT Techniques and Application to Intervention**		
Technique	Clinical Use	Intervention Application	Example
Handling	Hands used to support and assist movement (active or passive) from one position to another; active assisted movement is always encouraged	Use of hands: light touch, intermittent touch, or firm manual contacts to guide and assist with movement; also taught to caregivers	Caregivers taught to pick up, carry, and move individual from one position to next by incorporating encouragement of key movement components into motion: midline control, symmetry, weight shift, rotation, and dissociation.
Positioning	Used to provide alignment, comfort, support, prevent deformity, and provide readiness to support or enhance independent movement	Positioning for support is used to provide stability, alignment, and prevent deformity. Positioning is also used to promote optimal independent function or position from which movement can most likely occur.	Positioning of persons with hemiplegia with trunk and head in midline; both extremities forward and resting on tabletop; positioning of child on floor may be in side sit to encourage and assist in acquisition of transition to all fours for creeping.
Use of Adaptive Equipment	Used to provide postural support, prevent deformity, promote alignment, enhance function, and offer mobility; a common adjunct to intervention with children with neurological impairment	In addition to positional uses, equipment can be used dynamically to assist in movement control. Common uses include using the equipment to place the individual in a set position to enhance the opportunity for movement, to increase the possibility of desirable responses, to decrease the possibility of undesirable responses, or to control the instability and thereby limit the degrees of freedom of a given movement.	Can range from the simple towel roll under the scapula to promote scapular protraction for reaching to the complex, such as powered mobility. Examples include adapted tricycles, switch toys, seating inserts, toilet adaptations, standers, strollers, and wide ranges of pediatric wheelchairs. Equipment commonly used during dynamic movement, such as during therapy, include wedges, rolls, bolsters, benches, and gymnastic balls.
Key Points of Control	Parts of the body chosen by the therapist as optimal from which to guide the person's movement	Proximal key points of control include trunk, shoulders, and pelvis; distal points are hands and feet (less frequently used)	Guide from the scapula or the pelvis to protract the extremity in preparation for a movement. The more proximal the therapist's guiding hands, the more control the therapist has, and less is given to the mover; more distal key points of control give more control to the mover.

TABLE 6–5	**Summary of NDT Techniques and Application to Intervention**		
Technique	Clinical Use	Intervention Application	Example
Facilitating Transitional Movement	Facilitation of key movement components during active transitional movement	Facilitation of antigravity control, weight bearing, weight shifting; responses to movement such as automatic postural responses, rotation, and dissociation	Used clinically most often to assist with weight shift in preparation for movement; movement is guided once the weight-bearing body part is stable allowing for the weight shift to be followed by movement of the body segment.
Use of Sensory Input	Voluntary movement control is facilitated through use of proprioceptive inputs, exteroceptive inputs, and visual, vestibular, and verbal inputs	Proprioceptive inputs include weight bearing, approximation, stretching and traction, and tapping. Exteroceptive inputs include manual guidance, therapeutic use of hands. Movement stimulates vestibular system and vision; verbal inputs are used for motor learning.	Handling, guided movements, use of visual demonstration and verbal feedback, use of movement to stimulate the vestibular system (with and without equipment).
Motor Learning Strategies	Active movement is encouraged; practice, repetition, feedback, use of functional activities	Use of variable practice and problem solving in natural environments promotes motor learning.	Intervention takes place within environmental context: home, school, and community

Sources. Information compiled from multiple sources. See main text for details and references.

of motion) or as offered by a support (thorough postural support, manual support, or equipment). Assumptions underlying a task-oriented approach can be summarized as follows:

- Normal, functional movement emerges as an interaction among many systems, each contributing its own aspect of control.
- Movement is organized around a behavioral goal, constrained by the environment.
- Movement problems, as demonstrated in abnormal motor control, result from impairments within one or more of the systems controlling movement. The movement that is observed in the individual with neurological dysfunction emerges from the best mix of the systems remaining and able to participate in movement production. This means that the movement patterns that are observed are not just a result of the lesion itself but also of the efforts of the remaining systems to compensate for the damage and that continue to be functional. The compensatory strategy developed by the individual may or may not be optimal and efficient (Shumway-Cook and Woollacott, 2001).

These assumptions suggest that when training movement control, it is essential to work on identifiable functional tasks rather than on movement patterns for movement's sake alone. A task-oriented approach to intervention assumes that individuals learn by attempting to solve the problems inherent in a functional task rather than by repetitively practicing "normal" patterns of movement. Individuals are then guided in learning a variety of ways to solve the task goal so that the carryover between different environmental contexts can occur (Flinn, 1995). A task-oriented approach uses a multi-faceted approach to the clinical management of the individual with movement control problems. In order to apply this approach, a method for task analysis is necessary.

Example

It is important to remember the individual nature of functional task solution. In the example, getting out of bed, there are multiple solutions and strategies that could be effectively used to get out of bed. The learner can try this by observing different individuals within different environments, with different types of beds, and how many different styles of getting out of bed are observable. Skilled movement behavior is defined by the ability to adapt the movements used to achieve the goal of the task consistently and efficiently across a wide variety of environments. An individual is not considered functionally independent if he or she can get out of only one type of bed or out of a bed oriented in only one way in a room!

The goal of retraining at the functional task level focuses on having patients/clients successfully practice the performance of a wide collection of functional tasks in a variety of contexts. Analysis of patient performance on the functional level focuses on the ability of the individual to perform essential tasks and activities.

This task-oriented approach looks at and treats motor behavior by focusing on three levels: functional abilities, a description of the strategies used to accomplish functional skills, and recognition of the underlying impairments that constrain the functional movement. Intervention can be targeted at all three levels. This approach can integrate functional training, sensorimotor techniques when appropriate, and motor learning. Table 6–6 offers a helpful, concise worksheet for clinicians to use during task analysis and in the practice of this learning experience.

■ *Purpose*

The purpose of this exercise is to offer the learner an opportunity to practice performing functional task analyses.

■ *Materials*

None.

■ *Instructions*

Chose a new task to teach a partner. Using Table 6–6, go through all the steps involved in task analysis. Afterward, ask your partner to critique the learning experience. Switch roles, and repeat. Chose a clinically applicable task such as a mobility task (transferring, a gait task, rolling, bed mobility), a self-care task (dressing, feeding, hygiene), or a work or leisure task (gardening or performing a home repair). Practice teaching the tasks to each other and using Table 6–6 to become proficient at task analysis.

For each task, have a dialogue with your partner (role-playing the part of the patient), and write a functional goal. All functional goals should contain the following elements: who will do what, under what conditions, how well, and by when.

_____

_____

_____

_____

_____

_____

_____

_____

_____

_____

_____

Learning Experience Three: Functional Training

Functional training, as an intervention approach, has developed from a practical application of motor control and motor learning knowledge, therapeutic exercise application, motor development, and a task-oriented approach to movement reeducation. Functional training in the purest sense is a method of retraining the movement system, using repetitive practice of functional tasks in an attempt to establish or reestablish the individual's ability to perform activities of daily living (Umphred et al, 2001). Functional training focuses on using a variety of different motor skills necessary for everyday life, including transitions between and within postures; skills needed for activities of daily living, such as reaching, lifting, and turning; and skills necessary for instrumental activities of daily living, such as performing simple home repair and engaging in meaningful hobbies and valuable work. It also focuses on showing each individual how to adapt different movements in order to respond to changing environmental demands (O'Sullivan, 2001). Functional training can be implemented once the clinician has identified the individual's functional limitations. Guided by the question, " What tasks of value to the patient can he/she do and not do?" identified functional tasks can be performed and practiced. It is essentially important that the choice of functional task goals be centered around the activities that are meaningful and valuable to the individual

TABLE 6–6	**A Clinical Strategy for Using Task Analysis in Patient Instruction and Observation**	
Step	Main Decision/Action	Key Aspects

Step 1	Identify task	* Specify goal and subgoals
		* Gather critical information about:
		  • Environment
		  • Individual mover
		  • Prerequisite skills needed
		  • Expectations of outcome

Step 2	Develop a strategy to teach or observe task	* Develop strategy to make up for deficits identified in previous step * Plan any intervention strategy to optimize the individual task-environment interaction

Step 3	Effect the strategy, and analyze the task	* Observe the performance of the individual
		* Make any appropriate comparison
		* Analyze
		* Record what happened:
		  • What was the outcome of the attempt?
		  • What was the approach?
		  • What was the effect of the movement solution?

Step 4	Practice	* Identify missing components * Explanation: clear goal identification * Instruction * Feedback * Manual guidance * Ongoing reevaluation * Encourage flexibility
Step 5	Evaluate observations	* Compare expectations with outcome * Provide feedback and assist learner in generating plan for next attempt
Step 6	Transfer of training	* Give opportunity to practice in varying contexts * Offer consistency and variability of practice * Assist organization of self-monitored practice * Involve caregivers, relatives, and staff

Adapted from Arend and Higgins, 1976; Craik and Oatis, 1995; Bennett and Karnes, 1998.

patient/client. Occupation in meaningful activity is the cornerstone of wellness.

The main focus on functional training is the correction of functional limitations. A functional limitation is a restriction of the ability to perform, at the level of the whole person, a physical action, activity, or task, in an efficient, typically expected, or competent manner (APTA, 2001). A crucial next step is the prioritizing of what systems or activities the patient really needs to change and choosing the activities to emphasize during functional training. In an attempt to help individuals achieve their potential for movement and function, treatment/intervention is directed toward the primary and secondary impairments, movement problems, and the functional limitations that may contribute to disability. For patients with neurological disorders, this intervention process is threefold: movement reeducation, elimination or reduction of impairments, and functional training (see text). Activities incorporating task-oriented training are more motivating and goal-directed for the individual. The most contemporary approach combines functional activities into task-oriented training. This approach integrates dynamic systems theory with motor learning theory. It is based on the theory that the systems within the central nervous system are organized primarily to control function (Reed, 1982). Its central theme is that the interacting subsystems contributing to the production of movement are organized around essential functional movement tasks and the environment within which the task is performed. Its emphasis is on the use of functional tasks and contexts in intervention, drawing from a systems model of motor control.

There are several texts that describe this approach

to functional retraining for persons with neurological impairment of function (Carr and Shepherd, 1987, 1998; Palmer and Toms, 1992; Ryerson and Levit, 1997). The clinician is a facilitator, keeping physically guided movements to a minimum so that the individual is encouraged and supported to be an active participant in solving unique movement problems. This approach offers an insightful perspective on motor education and reeducation, offering specific suggestions on how to break down common functional movement tasks into component parts.

On a practical note, individuals with deficits in movement control present with both unique and variable patterns of functional limitations. Underlying impairments (presence of and significance of) must be linked to functional performance. Functional limitations may vary by the task, the environment, and the individual. A conceptual framework for intervention allows different postures, activities, and treatment techniques to be classified according to function. The terms mobility, stability, controlled mobility, and skill can be used in an easily applicable functional training intervention framework (O'Sullivan and Schmitz 2001). Functional movement requires that the *relative distribution* of stability and mobility be continuously adapted and changed. The most stable body part or segment needs some component of mobility for dynamic stability, and the most mobile body part needs some component of stability for the smooth grading of movement. (Tscharnuter, 1993) Functional movement reflects this intricate relationship between mobility and stability. Treatment suggestions include progression through increasingly difficult postures and activities, and intervention techniques are used to assist with movement as active voluntary control emerges. In a functional training approach and in functional mobility training, the therapist or assistant guides the patient in performing and practicing tasks that are relevant and important for optimum functional performance for that individual.

▪ *Purpose*

The purpose of this exercise is to offer the learner an opportunity to integrate the use of manual techniques and task analyses into a holistic approach intended to help the individual gain or regain functional movement.

▪ *Materials*

Materials found within a natural environmental setting for any individual.

▪ *Instructions*

In the learning laboratory setting, practice using all the approaches depicted in the figures in this chapter in the main text. Practice your hand placement, the amount of control you have as the clinician as compared with the amount of active control you are giving your partner who is acting in the role of a patient. Further suggestions for practice can be found in the cited texts, which offer a plethora of pictures demonstrating functional training in rehabilitation (Carr and Shepherd, 1998; O'Sullivan and Schmitz, 2001 text and laboratory manual; Palmer and Toms, 1992; Ryerson and Levit, 1997). The cases at the end of the text chapter also contain many photographs of patient intervention that can be perused and practiced at this time.

Review Questions

1. What is the relationship between theoretical advances and models of clinical practice?

2. What are the key contributions of the reflex theory and the hierarchical theory, and how did these early theories add to an understanding of motor behavior?

3. What are the guiding principles behind the dynamic systems approach to intervention with the patient/client with a neurological impairment?

4. What is meant by the "sensorimotor" approach to treatment? Describe some useful intervention tools derived from this approach.

5. What are the key intervention concepts central to proprioceptive neuromuscular facilitation? Describe some of the common intervention techniques offered by this approach.

6. What are the key concepts central to neurodevelopmental treatment? Describe some of the common techniques offered by this approach.

7. What were the main contributions of Brunnstrom's movement theory to the treatment of patients with hemiplegia? Describe the stages of recovery and synergy patterns as commonly observed in patients with hemiplegia.

_____

_____

_____

_____

8. What were the key treatment concepts central to the neurophysiological approach as proposed by Margaret Rood? Describe some of the common treatment techniques offered by this approach.

_____

_____

_____

_____

9. What are the key concepts central to sensory integration as a frame of reference? How would you incorporate some of these principles into the clinical management of a person with a neurological disorder?

_____

_____

_____

_____

10. When are sensorimotor techniques useful as part of an integrated approach to a patient's treatment?

_____

_____

_____

_____

11. How can a task-oriented model of intervention be applied to the evaluation and treatment of patients/clients with neurological disorders?

_____

_____

_____

_____

12. How would you perform an effective task analysis?

_____

_____

_____

_____

13. Describe what is meant by all the different types of strategies demonstrated by an individual during performance of a movement: movement strategies, sensory strategies, cognitive and perceptual strategies, compensatory strategies, age-related strategy changes.

_____

_____

_____

_____

14. What is meant by recovery versus compensation and appropriate versus undesirable compensation strategies, and what are the key differences in these terms?

_____

_____

_____

_____

15. What is meant by impairment? List some of the common impairments in individuals with a neurological disorder.

_____

_____

_____

_____

16. How would you as a clinician apply the task-oriented model to the management of an individual with a neurological disorder?

_____

_____

_____

_____

17. How would you apply a functional training approach to intervention with an individual with a neurological disorder?

_____

_____

_____

_____

18. What would be some useful strategies for improving functional mobility, such as mobility, stability, controlled mobility, and skill?

_____

_____

_____

_____

19. What is meant by functional limitation (activity limitation) and functional goals? Describe the clinical process used in intervening with an individual according to person-centered functional goals.

_____

_____

_____

_____

20. Why is it useful to adhere to an integrated approach in intervention with individuals with neurological impairment presenting at any age?

_____

_____

_____

_____

Clinical Management of the Primary Neuromuscular Impairments That Interfere With Functional Movement

7

This chapter of both the workbook and the text is the first of four clinical management chapters; this chapter focuses on the primary neuromuscular impairments that typically accompany neurological dysfunction. Damage to the central nervous system is accompanied by both positive and negative features. The text discusses at length the clinical management of the following commonly encountered impairments: muscular weakness; abnormal muscle tone, including abnormally low and abnormally high muscle tone; coordination problems, including problems with muscle activation, sequencing, and timing; and interference from involuntary movements, including dystonia, tremor, associated movements, and athetoid or choreiform movements. Figures and case studies give examples of effective intervention approaches for the management of the common movement dilemmas contributed to by some of these impairments.

Functional training and enablement are the cornerstones of the interventions described. The nature of the functional movement problem in individuals with a neurological impairment is a complex issue with many contributing variables, least of which is not the uniqueness of each individual. Abnormal patterns of movement are no longer considered to be purely evidence of abnormal muscle tone or disinhibited lower centers. Rather, the observed abnormal patterns of movement may perhaps be explained, at least clinically, as a functional adaptation to motor performance that becomes apparent when an individual attempts to move in the presence of muscle weakness and imbalance between stronger and weaker muscle groups. When an individual with a brain injury attempts a purposeful action, the movement pattern that emerges reflects the *best* that can be done *under the circumstances*, given the state of

both the neural and musculoskeletal systems and the dynamic possibilities inherent in the linkages between all of the subsystems involved in movement production and control (Carr and Shepherd, 1998). The movements that emerge may or may not be distorted.

Problem-solving clinicians need to identify first what factor or factors seem to interfere most with motor performance. Encouraging the patient/client to be active seems to be a critical factor. Engaging the individual in meaningful, occupational-embedded tasks is crucial for success. Neurological rehabilitation should begin early and be active (Carr and Shepherd, 1987, 1998; Richards et al, 1991) Based on the current knowledge available, Carr and Shepherd (1998) offer the following recommendations for rehabilitation intervention when working with patients with a neurological disorder who present with movement problems complicated by abnormal force generation:

- Intensive training and practice, including task-related exercise, directed at eliciting muscle activity, controlling force generation and synergistic muscle activity, and strengthening muscles.
- Preserving length and flexibility of all tissues.

Please see text for full details.

Active Learning Experiences

Learning Experience One: Task Analysis of Common Functional Activities

As detailed in the previous chapter, the ability to analyze how a task is executed is a crucial skill needed for teaching the safe and successful performance of functional activities.

▪ Purpose

The purpose of this exercise is to offer the learner an opportunity to practice task analysis of common functional activities.

▪ Materials

Materials found within naturally occurring environments as used in the example and in suggested task activities: bed, bed covers, a variety of different chairs.

▪ Instructions

Using the example below as a model, perform the following functional activities and perform a task analysis of that movement. Use the space below each suggested activity to list each step of the task, as you observe a partner perform each task. After doing the task analyses, teach each component as well as the whole task to a partner.

Example

A frequent problem reported by individuals with movement disorders is difficulty turning over and getting out of bed. This complex sequential motor skill has many components. The following illustrates how a clinician could analyze this task for retraining (Morris, 2000):

1. Throwing back the bed covers
2. Shifting the pelvis toward the center of the bed so that, when the turn is completed, the body is not too close to the edge
3. Turning the head
4. Bringing the arm across the body in the direction of the roll or turn
5. Swinging the legs over the edge
6. Pushing up
7. Adjusting postural alignment to sit upright

▪ Suggested Task One

Lying down in bed from sitting on the edge of the bed

▪ Suggested Task Two

Getting up from a chair to standing

▪ Suggested Task Three

Standing up from supine on the floor

Learning Experience Two: Clinical Intervention Practice

At the end of every chapter in Part Two of the text, there are adult and child case studies. These case studies illustrate the key concepts covered in that chapter. In addition, they offer opportunities for learners to partner or work in small groups as a role-playing activity.

▪ Purpose

The purpose of this exercise is to offer the learner an opportunity to practice several different skills: clinical reasoning, clinician-client interaction and com-munication, observation skills, assessment techniques, and intervention techniques

▪ Materials

Material required to practice in a clinical laboratory setting the case studies presented at the end of the text chapter. See text for reference.

▪ Instructions

Divide into small groups (three or four is optimal). Role-play each of the three case studies at the end of this chapter in the text. One student is the patient, another is the therapist or assistant, and the remaining one or two persons observe the intervention and critique. Discuss in small groups, and summarize for the instructor.

Review Questions

1. Define and describe the primary neuromuscular impairments associated with neurological dysfunction: muscle weakness, abnormalities of muscle tone, coordination problems, interference from involuntary movements.

_____

_____

_____

_____

2. What is the difference between a positive and a negative feature of brain damage? Give an example of each.

_____

_____

_____

_____

3. What is the difference between a primary and secondary impairment? Give an example of each. What kind of an impact on functional performance can impairment have?

_____

_____

_____

_____

4. What is muscular weakness? How does it develop as a result of upper motor neuron pathology? What are some of the clinical consequences of this weakness?

_____

_____

_____

_____

5. What is muscle tone?

_____

_____

_____

_____

6. What are hypotonia and flaccidity? What are the clinical signs associated with abnormally low muscle tone, and how can abnormally low muscle tone affect movement control?

_____

_____

_____

_____

7. What are the common clinical problems, functional impairments, and therapy goals most appropriate for the individual presenting with hypotonia?

_____

_____

_____

_____

8. Differentiate between spasticity and stiffness. What are the clinical signs associated with spasticity, and how can spasticity affect movement control?

_____

_____

_____

_____

9. What are some of the main therapeutic interventions for the clinical management of spasticity? How do these interventions attempt to decrease the influence of this symptom of disordered motor control and subsequently improve voluntary movement?

_____

_____

_____

_____

10. What are the common clinical problems, functional impairments, and therapy goals of the individual presenting with hypertonicity?

_____

_____

_____

_____

11. What is rigidity, and what are the different types of rigidity: decerebrate, decorticate, cogwheel, and lead pipe? What pathological conditions are associated with which types of rigidity?

_____

_____

_____

_____

12. What are some of the main therapeutic interventions for the clinical management of rigidity, directed to decrease the influence of this symptom of disordered motor control on movement?

_____

_____

_____

_____

13. Describe the impairments of uncoordinated movement, and describe what is meant by problems with muscle activation, sequencing, and timing.

_____

_____

_____

_____

14. What are some of the main therapeutic interventions for the clinical management of uncoordinated movement, directed to decrease the influence of this symptom of disordered motor control on movement?

_____

_____

_____

_____

15. Define and describe the involuntary movements: dystonia, tremor, associated movements, athetoid or choreiform movements. What are their clinical effects on movement control?

_____

_____

_____

_____

16. What are some of the main therapeutic interventions for the clinical management of involuntary movement, directed to decrease the influence of this symptom of disordered motor control on movement?

_____

_____

_____

_____

17. What are the common clinical problems, functional impairments, and therapy goals of the individual presenting with dystonia?

_____

_____

_____

_____

18. What are the key components of a functional, task-related approach to intervention with an individual who has functional movement problem caused by neurological dysfunction?

_____

_____

_____

_____

19. Guided by case study examples, describe the main intervention strategies and techniques used for the following three functional movement disorders: patient with hemiplegia following a stroke, during the flaccid and spastic phase; patient with parkinsonian rigidity and movement coordination difficulties; patient with developmental disorder, dystonia, and involuntary movements.

_____

_____

_____

_____

Management of Disorders of Postural Control and Balance

Catherine Emery, MS, OTR/L, BCN

The ability to keep the body steady while engaged in activities that use the limbs is critical to functional independence. Control of posture provides the stable base from which balance is achieved in a variety of body positions, whether the body is still, preparing to move, or preparing to stop (Wade and Jones, 1997). There are many tasks involved within the intricacies and complexities of the postural control and balance systems. These systems are involved in recovery from instability *as well as* the ability to anticipate and move to avoid instability (Shumway-Cook and Woollacott, 2001). Stability develops from postural adjustments made through the postural control systems (Wade and Jones, 1997). These adjustments serve to reduce or eliminate a displacement of the center of gravity in order to allow safe movement (Frank and Earl, 1990).

To maintain this stability, coordinated muscle contractions must occur around the joints. This coordination must be flexible enough to allow for adjustment to changes in the environment. Co-contraction needs to occur continuously and be somewhat removed from voluntary suppression (Littell, 1990). In other words, it is important to have the muscles that stabilize the joints working at all times in order to keep the body upright. It is equally important to limit the ability of the conscious brain to reduce this action. Many small corrective muscle actions are made to prevent falling, whether the body position is standing quietly; doing the simplest movement, such as waving to a friend; or engaging in complex motions, like those required when trying to regain balance after a slip on an icy surface (Cohen, 1999). An additional key element of postural control is

orientation—defined as keeping the body segments in an appropriate relationship with each other and the environment in order to complete functional tasks. An important goal of postural control is to provide stability to the sensory and motor systems. This stability optimizes the influx of sensory information while moving (Wade and Jones, 1997).

Active Learning Experiences

Learning Experience One: Awareness of the Motor Strategies Used as Postural Control Recovery Strategies

Researchers (Horak and Nashner, 1986) have identified automatic movements used to keep the center of motion over the base of support. The responses are stereotypical; they match the direction and degree of the challenge given (Umphred, 2001). For example, if a person is pushed to the right side, the automatic response is a shift to the left to reestablish midline. The harder the destabilizing challenge, the greater the movement to realign the body, as body segments are activated to oppose the reaction forces (Frank and Earl, 1990). Environmental features, true to the systems model, do have an influence on the production of strategies; in a new environment, a person may take a step earlier than might have happened in a more familiar, less anxiety-provoking situation.

Increasingly, the contribution of trunk and hip input is being studied as more important than lower leg input to shaping the balance strategy (Allum et al, 1998). These postural adjustments serve to minimize the displacement of the center of gravity in order to allow safe and efficient voluntary movement (Frank and Earl, 1990). Interestingly, this selection of muscles is presumed to be shaped by vestibular input developed in early infancy to prevent falls (Allum et al, 1990).

▪ Purpose

The purpose of this exercise is to offer the learner an opportunity to feel the various motor recovery strategies used to regain postural control and balance. Several activities are described.

▪ Materials

For this activity, the learner is encouraged to be outside, if possible, near a curb.

▪ Instructions

Walk along a raised curb, focusing on each step taken. Notice how the body moves when imbalance occurs. Does movement at the ankles happen more than at the hips?

_____

_____

Now cross the same length of raised curb, but place each foot in front of the other heel-to-toe. How does this change the movements for recovery?

_____

_____

Again, walk across the curb, being sure not to watch the feet, and focus on a point in the distance at eye level. Note how the body moves in its attempts to maintain posture and balance.

_____

_____

Learning Experience Two: Sensory Strategy Assessment

Sensory strategies are ways of organizing sensory input to alert the motor systems to make changes to the plan or execution of movement. Reducing the amount of conflicting sensory input and coordinat-

ing sensory information with motor aspects of postural control are the methods of organization that seem to be used. Effective postural control requires the ability to generate forces to control the body's position in space and to know where the body is in space and whether it is moving (Shumway-Cook and Woollacott, 2001). All the sensory systems contribute to maintaining postural control in the absence of challenges.

In the presence of challenges, each sensory system appears to take on a different role in correcting balance. This is due in part to the limitation of each system: the visual system cannot distinguish between body movement and environmental movement without vestibular input. Likewise, the vestibular system cannot distinguish head movement, for instance a head nod, from combined head and body movement, such as a forward bow, without contributions from the proprioceptors (Umphred, 2001). When the brain becomes aware of abnormal signals, the normal sensory input gains importance for position in space to be perceived accurately (Umphred, 2001). When the brain is unable to determine which system is providing erroneous input, an attempt is made to decrease input in order to evaluate each system. For example, vertigo (a sense of movement when there is no actual movement) is sometimes experienced after rising to a standing position. Closing the eyes can reduce the discomfort it creates, effectively reducing the sensory input being gathered by an overwhelmed system.

Example

Remember the strategies used when visiting the amusement park during summer vacation. As the merry-go-round rotates, the riders focus on one spot in order to reduce the risk of vomiting as they disembark. Another instance where input is reduced is during ice-skating or skiing activities. Muscles are tensed to give an increased experience of control as well as to reduce the extraneous movement felt.

The sensory strategies seem to be selected in a hierarchy to better ensure that the appropriate sense is selected for the task (Shumway-Cook and Woollacott, 2001). The selection process also varies based on age, the task at hand, and the context in which the task is occurring.

▪ Purpose

The purpose of this exercise is to offer the learner an opportunity to experience the body's reliance on somatosensory information to guide movement and provide postural control.

▪ Materials

Plastic safety glasses, skin lotion or petroleum jelly, beanbag chair, overhead object to reach for (i.e., cabinet).

▪ Instructions

Cover a pair of plastic safety glasses with lotion or petroleum jelly. Put them on, and walk steadily down an unfamiliar path. What are the segments of the body doing in this condition of simulated impairment?

_____

_____

_____

_____

What new input does the body become more aware of?

_____

_____

_____

_____

What is your speed of movement?

_____

_____

_____

_____

Next, step on a beanbag chair, and reach into a cabinet overhead. What does the body do to compensate for the imprecise somatosensory input?

_____

_____

_____

_____

Review Questions

1. What is postural control?

_____

_____

_____

_____

2. What is balance?

_____

_____

_____

_____

3. What are postural adjustments? When are they used?

_____

_____

_____

_____

4. What are postural preparations? When are they used?

_____

_____

_____

_____

5. What are postural accompaniments? When are they used?

_____

_____

_____

_____

6. What are the theoretical models used to explain the neural control of posture and balance?

_____

_____

_____

_____

7. Name the righting reactions. What is their relationship to the development of an awareness of gravity?

_____

_____

_____

_____

8. What are equilibrium reactions? What is their relationship to the development of motor milestones?

_____

_____

_____

_____

9. What are orienting reactions? Explain their role in development of postural control and balance.

_____

_____

_____

_____

10. What is head control? How does it contribute to movement?

_____

_____

_____

_____

11. How does postural sway influence trunk control development?

_____

_____

_____

_____

12. Give at least one example of a musculoskeletal limitation that contributes to postural instability.

_____

_____

_____

_____

13. Identify and explain the three neuromuscular factors that contribute to the organization of muscle forces for postural control.

_____

_____

_____

_____

14. What are the three primary systems whose input directly affects postural control and balance?

_____

_____

_____

_____

15. What is the importance of vision to humans? What are some implications for function of this strong sensory reliance?

_____

_____

_____

_____

16. Explain the three visual projection areas. What is their role in vision and perception?

_____

_____

_____

_____

17. What is the difference between focal and ambient vision?

_____

_____

_____

_____

18. What are the major anatomical structures of the vestibular system? Explain their role in awareness of movement.

_____

_____

_____

_____

19. What is the importance of the vestibular structures? What are the functional implications of their input for postural control and balance?

_____

_____

_____

_____

20. What are the differences between central and peripheral vestibular disorders?

_____

_____

_____

_____

21. What is the definition of vestibular-ocular reflex?

_____

_____

_____

_____

22. What are the major anatomical structures of the peripheral system that are related to postural control and balance? Explain their role in awareness of movement.

_____

_____

_____

_____

23. What is perception?

_____

_____

_____

_____

24. What is the difference between body image and body scheme? What are their respective roles in postural control and balance?

_____

_____

_____

_____

25. What are the definitions of laterality and directionality?

_____

_____

_____

_____

26. How do cognitive mechanisms influence postural control and balance and treatment of imbalance?

_____

_____

_____

_____

27. What are the strategies used by the sensory system for postural stability and balance?

_____

_____

_____

_____

28. What is the definition of vertigo?

_____

_____

_____

_____

29. Define the ankle strategy of postural recovery. When is it mostly used to control posture and balance?

_____

_____

_____

_____

30. Define the hip strategy of postural recovery. When is it mostly used to control posture and balance?

_____

_____

_____

_____

31. Define the stepping strategy of postural recovery. When is it mostly used to control posture and balance?

_____

_____

_____

_____

32. What are the differences between controlled movement and skilled movement?

_____

_____

_____

_____

33. What is reactive and anticipatory control?

_____

_____

_____

_____

34. What are the major challenges to developing postural control in early development?

_____

_____

_____

_____

35. What are the major challenges to developing postural control in childhood?

_____

_____

_____

_____

36. What are the major challenges to developing postural control in adolescence?

_____

_____

_____

_____

37. What are the major challenges to developing postural control in adulthood?

_____

_____

_____

_____

38. Identify the musculoskeletal changes that occur with age. How do they affect postural control and balance?

_____

_____

_____

_____

39. What are the neuromuscular changes that occur with age? How do they affect postural control and balance?

_____

_____

_____

_____

40. What are several sensory changes that occur with age? How do they affect postural control and balance?

_____

_____

_____

_____

41. What cognitive changes result from aging? How do they affect postural control and balance?

_____

_____

_____

_____

42. What are some functional balance assessments? What is their role in assessing postural instability or imbalance?

_____

_____

_____

_____

43. What are some assessments of balance systems? What is their role in determining the factors causing postural instability or imbalance?

_____

_____

_____

_____

44. What are the differences between the impairment, strategy, and functional levels of intervention for postural stability and balance problems?

_____

_____

_____

_____

45. What are some techniques for remediation of balance dysfunction at the impairment level?

_____

_____

_____

_____

46. What are some techniques for remediation of balance dysfunction at the strategy level?

_____

_____

_____

_____

47. What is the definition of the functional level of task performance? Explain the importance of context in addressing postural and balance dysfunction.

_____

_____

_____

_____

Management of the Impaired Upper Extremity

Doré Blanchet, MS, OTR/L

Many systems work together to allow individuals to use their arms and hands to interact with the environment. The importance of the sensory systems such as vision, proprioception, and touch help prepare the individual to reach, to adapt to changes in the environment, and to refine the delicate in-hand manipulation skills that are often performed without much thought. Through the development of proximal stability in weight-bearing positions as an infant and sensory exploration of objects in the environment, the individual gains the freedom to eventually engage in dynamic interactions with the environment, using his or her upper extremity. These interactions can be as simple as brushing one's teeth or as complex as performing a Mozart violin concerto. The upper extremity functions of regard, reach, grasp, manipulation, and release cannot be achieved without coordination of multiple body systems and the volition of the individual. Context, the role of the environment, and the actual task that is being performed have a great impact on the outcome and the ability to reach.

Active Learning Experiences

Learning Experience One: The Importance of Proprioception in Reach*

Proprioceptive input, received through joint receptors, Golgi tendon organs, and muscle spindles, provides the information that tells the movement system how to position the extremity in space by acti-

vating certain muscles. "The major sense working alongside vision is this proprioceptive sense, providing information about movements and position of the body and its parts" (Sugden, 1990 p. 133). An example of proprioceptive input and vision working together can be observed in catching a ball, in which vision provides the information concerning the object, speed, and trajectory, and the proprioceptive system provides the information needed to position the upper extremity in order to catch the ball (Sugden, 1990).

■ **Purpose**

The following activity described by Leonard (1998) is intended to help the learner to experience a demonstrated role of proprioceptive input during reach.

■ **Materials**

A vibrator.

■ **Instructions**

Divide into pairs. One partner closes both eyes and extends one arm away from his or her body. With eyes closed, the individual touches his or her own nose. Repeat this two times. Then, the other member of the pair vibrates the individual's triceps tendon for a few moments, with the individual's eyes closed and arm extended. Now the individual again tries to touch his or her own nose while keeping the eyes shut. Discuss the following questions:

---

* Adapted from Leanord,1998, with permission from Elsevier.

1. What happened following vibration of the tendon?

_____

_____

2. Why do you think this occurred?

_____

_____

3. Which systems eventually recognize your error?

_____

_____

_____

Learning Experience Two: The Importance of Posture in Shoulder Alignment and Reach

For patients/clients who present with a neurological impairment, poor postural alignment over time can lead to numerous difficulties with reach and grasp. Secondary impairments of contracture, weakness, and pain are just some of the common complications that are observed.

▪ Purpose

The following activity will allow the learner to simulate some of the common postures observed in the client with a neurological disorder and to understand the effect these postures have on reach.

▪ Materials

None.

▪ Instructions

For this activity, the learners should work in pairs and wear a tank top or clothing that allows visualization of the shoulder girdle. Have a member of each pair assume the postures listed below. Record the position of the scapula and humerus. Then have the learner maintain this posture and try to reach for something just above eye level and then maintain his or her grasp. Have the learner describe how this felt. Talk about the components of regard, reach, grasp, and release while maintaining these postures.

1. Excessive trunk flexion, posterior pelvic tilt, neck flexion

_____

_____

_____

_____

2. Excessive trunk flexion, posterior pelvic tilt, shoulder elevation, neck hyperextension

_____

_____

_____

_____

3. Excessive trunk extension, anterior pelvic tilt

_____

_____

_____

_____

4. Lateral trunk flexion on the reaching side

_____

_____

_____

_____

5. Trunk flexion with lateral flexion on the reaching side

_____

_____

_____

_____

Learning Experience Three: How the Properties of the Task Affect Reach and Grasp Movement

The speed and movements that encompass the ability to reach depend largely on the goal of the reaching task (Shumway-Cook and Woollacott, 2001). The velocity of arm movements when reaching toward an object changes based on the nature of the task, the properties of the object, and the environmental context. For example, when an individual reaches to grasp a small glass ornament, the velocity of the reach will be much slower than when picking up keys from a table. Reaching movements could also change based on the environmental context, such as performing the above tasks while rushing out the door late for a class.

▪ Purpose

The purpose of this exercise is to offer the learner an opportunity to examine and discuss how the properties of the task affect reach and grasp movements.

▪ Materials

A ring stacker with rings, a quarter and coin bank, a pencil and paper.

▪ Instructions

For this activity, divide into pairs. Perform the following activities; observe the patterns of reach, grasp, manipulation, and release; and discuss. Use the following questions to guide the observation and discussion. How did the task change the properties of regard, reach, grasp, manipulation, and release? When did anticipatory hand shaping occur? Note your discussion comments after each activity.

1. Place three rings, the quarter, and the pencil in a row on the table. Have a partner pick these items up and set them down. Observe the patterns of regard, reach, grasp, manipulation, and release. Answer the discussion questions.

_____

_____

_____

_____

_____

_____

_____

_____

2. Place the ring stacker next to the rings, the bank next to the coin, and the paper next to the pencil. Now observe your partner place the rings on the stacker, put the coin in the bank, and write his or her name on the piece of paper. Observe the patterns of regard, reach, grasp, manipulation, and release. Answer the discussion questions.

_____

_____

_____

_____

_____

_____

_____

_____

Review Questions

1. What are the some of the upper extremity functional tasks of an infant, child, and adult?

2. What is the function of the somatosensory system during reach, grasp, manipulation, and release?

3. What is the function of the visual system during regard, reach, grasp, manipulation, and release?

4. What is the difference between power and precision grasp? List the components needed for each.

5. What are some of the everyday activities that use a power grasp and a precision grasp? List three examples for each.

6. What is the difference between a lateral pinch, a two-point pinch, and a three-point pinch? Give an example of how each pinch pattern is used.

7. What is the developmental progression of reach and grasp in the infant?

_____

_____

_____

_____

8. What is anticipatory control? What are the foundational skills needed to develop this?

_____

_____

_____

_____

9. What is haptic perception? Why is it important?

_____

_____

_____

_____

10. What are the components needed to develop in-hand manipulation skills? When do these typically begin to develop?

_____

_____

_____

_____

11. What are translation, shift, and rotation? When are these skills used?

_____

_____

_____

_____

12. What are some of the changes that occur with aging that affect regard, reach, grasp, manipulation, and release?

_____

_____

_____

_____

13. What are the functional limitations of the upper extremity due to weakness in relation to regard, reach, grasp, manipulation, and release?

_____

_____

_____

_____

14. What are the functional limitations of the upper extremity due to abnormal muscle tone in relation to regard, reach, grasp, manipulation, and release?

_____

_____

_____

_____

15. What are the functional limitations of the upper extremity due to incoordination in relation to regard, reach, grasp, manipulation, and release?

_____

_____

_____

_____

16. What are some of the common functional limitations of the upper extremity in the individual with cerebral palsy in relation to regard, reach, grasp, manipulation, and release?

_____

_____

_____

_____

17. What are some of the main therapeutic interventions for clinical management of upper extremity dysfunction in the individual with cerebral palsy?

_____

_____

_____

_____

18. What are some of the common functional limitations of the upper extremity in the individual with cerebrovascular accident in relation to regard, reach, grasp, manipulation, and release?

_____

_____

_____

_____

19. What are some of the main therapeutic interventions for clinical management of upper extremity dysfunction in the individual with cerebrovascular accident?

_____

_____

_____

_____

20. What are some of the common functional limitations of the upper extremity in the individual with Parkinson's disease in relation to regard, reach, grasp, manipulation, and release?

_____

_____

_____

_____

21. What are some of the main therapeutic interventions for clinical management of upper extremity dysfunction for the individual with Parkinson's disease?

_____

_____

_____

_____

10

Management of Impaired Lower Extremity Function

The tasks of the lower extremity are classified as weight-bearing or non–weight-bearing functional movement tasks, then further divided into common functional locomotor tasks: rolling, crawling and creeping; transfer tasks; and gait. An analysis of the movements required for successful execution of these common locomotor tasks can aid the clinician in problem solving for patients/clients experiencing difficulties with these tasks and in designing and carrying out an effective intervention strategy.

Active Learning Experiences

Learning Experience One: Analysis of Locomotor Tasks

Locomotion is defined as the process of moving from one place to another. Exactly how that is accomplished depends on several factors: the exact task to be done, the interaction of all the body subsystems that will perform the task, and the environment in which the task will take place (Cech and Martin, 1995). Locomotion solves a basic need of the individual: to transport the body from one location to another. Locomotion is a *variable* skill in that the movement form will differ, depending on the goal and the particular movement solution needed to meet that particular goal. Locomotion, or this task of moving through space, includes many forms of movement: rolling, crawling and creeping, walking, running, galloping, skipping, and hopping.

Locomotion is a skill that involves functional use of the lower extremities and of the arm and hand complex. The arm/hand complex is frequently used in support of the locomotor act or can be a vital component of the movement (Craik and Oatis, 1995).

■ Purpose

The purpose of this exercise is to offer the learner an opportunity to analyze while observing the locomotor tasks of rolling, sit-to-stand transfer, and walking. In addition, the learner can use these observational insights, with the table as a guide, to instruct an individual in the performance of each of those common functional locomotor tasks.

■ Materials

None.

■ Instructions

Using Tables 10–1, 10–2, and 10–3, practice the task analysis as described by observing a partner execute the following locomotion activities: rolling (Table 10–1), sit-to-stand transfer (Table 10–2), and walking (Table 10–3). Through role-playing, practice the way you would use this information to analyze the locomotor task and to train a patient/client in these three locomotor activities: rolling, sit-to-stand transfer, and walking.

TABLE 10–1	**Retraining Rolling**	

Functional Task: Rolling from supine to side lying, requiring a movement of the center of gravity from supine to side lying

Movement Initiation Possibilities	Transitional Movement Choices	Extremity Activity
• Upper trunk flexion and rotation	• Upper trunk initiation and lower trunk rotates to meet upper trunk	• Upper trunk initiation and upper extremity moves with trunk to assist
• Lower trunk extension and rotation	• Lower trunk initiation and upper trunk rotates to meet lower trunk	• Lower trunk initiation and lower extremity assists trunk movement
• Nonsegmental pattern with spine in neutral	• Nonsegmental initiation in which upper and lower trunk move together	• Nonsegmental initiation requiring trunk and extremities move together

Excerpted from Ryerson and Levit (1997), with permission from Elsevier.

▪ Rolling

Use Table 10–1 to guide analysis and training instruction.

_____

_____

_____

_____

_____

_____

_____

_____

▪ Sit-to-Stand Transfer

Use Table 10–2 to guide analysis and training instruction.

_____

_____

_____

_____

_____

_____

_____

_____

TABLE 10–2	**Sit-to-Stand Transfer**	

Functional Task: Moving from sitting with a wide base of support and low center of gravity to standing with a small base of support and high center of gravity. Starting position is one of sitting, upper trunk controlled over lower trunk, hips and knees in flexion, and ankles in slight dorsiflexion.

Phase	Task	Requirements of Task
1. Weight shift phase	Generation of forward momentum of upper body through forward flexion of the trunk	• Activation of erector spinae muscles, contracting eccentrically • Body is fairly stable
2. Beginning of rise (buttocks off the chair)	Transferring of momentum from upper body to total body, allowing a lift of the body	• Coactivation of hip and knee extensor muscles • Stability requirement is greatest during this phase
3. Lift or extension phase	Extension at hips and knees results in vertical movement of body	• Hip and knee extension, trunk extension, ankle postural control • Stability requirement less than in previous phase
4. Stabilization phase	Attain postural stability in new upright position	• Task-dependent motion is complete • Body stability in vertical is achieved

From Schenkman et al (1990) with permission of the American Physical Therapy Association and Shumway-Cook and Wollacott (2001), with permission from Lippincott, Williams & Wilkins.

TABLE 10–3   A Practical Guide to the Functional Requirements of Gait

Subphase	Functional Task	Joint Angle Requirement	Prime Muscular Force
Initial Contact	• Weight acceptance • Shock absorption	Ankle: 90° Knee: 3°–5° flexion Hip: 30° flexion	Tibialis anterior Quadriceps and hamstrings Gluteus maximus and medius
Loading	• Weight acceptance • Shock absorption	Ankle: 15° plantarflexion Knee: up to 15° flexion Hip: 30° flexion	Tibialis anterior Quadriceps Gluteus maximus
Midstance	• Single limb support	Ankle: from 15° plantarflexion to 15° dorsiflexion Knee: 5° flexion Hip: full extension	Gastrocnemius and soleus Gluteus maximus, medius, and minimus; tensor fascia lata
Terminal Stance	• Single limb support • Propulsion	Ankle: 15° dorsiflexion to 20° plantarflexion Knee: moves into full extension Hip: 10° extension	Gastrocnemius
Preswing	• Propulsion	Ankle: 20° plantarflexion Knee: 40° flexion Hip: 10° extension	Gastrocnemius Hip adductors Rectus femoris
Initial Swing	• Limb shortening for foot clearance	Ankle: to neutral dorsiflexion Knee: 40°–60° flexion Hip: from extension to 30° flexion	Tibialis anterior Quadriceps (controlling) Iliopsoas
Midswing	• Limb shortening for foot clearance • Generation of momentum	Ankle: neutral Knee: 60° flexion Hip: 30° flexion	Tibialis anterior Iliopsoas
Terminal Swing	• Limb advancement • Preparation for initial contact • Deceleration	Ankle: neutral Knee: to full extension Hip: 30° flexion	Tibialis anterior Gluteus maximus and hamstrings

Information compiled from Craik, R. L., & Oatis, C.A. (1995). Gait analysis: Theory and application. St. Louis: MO: Mosby; Perry, J. (1992). Gait analysis: Normal and pathological function. Thorofare, NJ: Slack Inc.: Pathokinesiology Department Physical Therapy Department. (1989). Observational gait analysis handbook. Downey, CA: The Professional Staff Association of Rancho Los Amigos Medical Center; Winter, D. A. (1985). Concerning the scientific basis for the diagnosis of pathological gait and for rehabilitation protocols. Physiotherapy Canada, 37, 245-252; and Winter, D. A. (1987). The biomechanics and motor control of human gait. Waterloo, Ontario: University of Waterloo Press.

Walking

Use Table 10–3 to guide analysis and training instruction.

_____

_____

_____

_____

_____

_____

Learning Experience Two: Observational Gait Analysis

Consistent with the emphasis on functionality in this text and workbook, it is imperative that clinicians also have an appreciation of the function of each of the eight subphases of gait so that observation, analysis, and intervention can be as accurate and meaningful as possible. A functional study of an individual's gait is performed by carefully assessing each phase of gait and the ability of the individual to meet the main three functional gait subtasks of limb loading, weight transfer, and limb advancement. Careful analysis of one joint at a time and one motion at a time will lead to a determination of contributing impairments and a practical clinical management plan.

▪ Purpose

It is amazing that an entire gait cycle is completed in little more than a second. Because gait occurs so rapidly with the subphases occurring in quick succession, it is important that students and clinicians have a method for observing. The following exercise offers the learner an opportunity to practice and refine an observational gait analysis strategy.

▪ Materials

This activity needs to be performed in a well-lit area devoid of obstacles, with a flat flooring surface, with the observed person either in bare feet or wearing comfortable shoes.

▪ Instructions

The following guidelines are offered:

1. Observe the individual walking in a well-lit area devoid of obstacles, either in bare feet or wearing comfortable shoes and using an assistive device, if prescribed.
2. Observation should be of several strides over a distance of several meters; the observer should stand at the middle of this distance in order to focus on typical walking and not on either the acceleration or deceleration portions of the walk.
3. Observe from a sagittal view and a frontal view, right and left sides, anterior and posterior.
4. Observe in a systematic fashion, starting at the head and neck and moving to the trunk, upper extremities, pelvis, hip, knee, and ankle/foot.

Use the following questions and format as a guide in performing an observational gait analysis.

Observational Gait Analysis

Sagittal Plane Analysis: Perform by viewing right and left sides.

Body Segment	Guiding Questions
Head, trunk, and arms	Does the head maintain a neutral position?
	Do the upper extremities swing rhythmically with the opposite lower extremities?
	Does the trunk rotate forward and backward with the swinging arm?
	Is there any excessive lean of the trunk either forward or backward, especially during early stance phase when weight is accepted?
Pelvis and hips	Does the pelvis rotate forward on the swinging side and backward with the stance side?
	As weight is accepted over the stance limb, does the hip continue to extend in support of the limb and in preparation for propulsion?
	During swing, does the hip flex smoothly forward in preparation for initial contact?
Knees	Is movement of the knee smooth or jerky as it moves through extension, flexion, extension, and then flexion again during stance?
	Does the knee appear to be stable as it accepts and loads weight?
	During swing, does the knee flex adequately for limb clearance?

Frontal Plane Analysis: Perform from both an anterior and a posterior view.

Feet and ankles	What does initial contact look like? Is it onto a heel strike or a foot flat? Is it quiet?
	During swing, does the foot dorsiflex adequately so that the foot clears the floor?
Head and trunk	Does the head face the frontal plane in midline?
	Is the trunk aligned in midline from the frontal plane, or is there any obvious asymmetry?
Pelvis and hips	Does the pelvis tilt down only slightly on the swinging side?
	Does there appear to be any excessive vertical displacement of the pelvis or hip (hip hike or vaulting)?
	Does hip extension stability appear to be adequate for weight acceptance and then propulsion?
	During swing, what does the path of the limb look like? Is there any excessive internal or external rotation or any sign of circumduction?
Knees	Is there any sign of excessive varus or valgus at the knees?
Feet and ankles	Does the foot and ankle complex appear to be stable during weight bearing?
	Is normal foot alignment maintained, or is the foot positioned in supination or pronation?

Sources: Information compiled from multiple sources. See main text for details and references.

Summarize your findings.

_____

_____

_____

_____

_____

_____

_____

_____

_____

Learning Experience Three: Task Analysis of Functional Subtasks of Gait

To help treat gait disturbances in the individual who has a neurological impairment, a model for task analysis is useful so that clinicians and students can discern with which part of the task during gait the patient is having difficulty: weight acceptance, single limb support, or limb advancement. A task-oriented approach is useful for training or retraining all locomotor activities, including gait. For example, patients with cerebral palsy or post-cerebrovascular accident will encounter difficulties with all three functional subtasks of gait, although patients with Parkinson's disease may have more difficulty with limb advancement than with weight acceptance or single limb support. Careful analysis can be used to aid in clinical decision making as the clinician seeks to answer key clinical questions.

▪ Purpose

The purpose of this learning experience is to illustrate the value of a task-oriented approach to the analysis and subsequent intervention for a gait disturbance as observed in an individual with a neurological impairment.

▪ Materials

Various assistive devices.

▪ Instructions

Observe your partner walking. Assess for demonstration/presence of the effectiveness of the main functional subtasks of gait: limb loading, weight transfer, and limb advancement. Take turns role-playing the following gait patterns seen commonly in clinical practice, and note the quality of the performance of these functional subtasks. For each clinical example, answer the following questions. Engage in a discussion of the impact of what you find upon assessment of that patient's locomotor function, and offer some intervention suggestions.

1. Patient with hemiplegic gait characterized by low trunk muscle tone, pelvic retraction, increased extension during stance, insufficient knee flexion during gait, and a foot drop due to anterior tibialis paralysis.
   • With which functional subtasks of gait is this individual having difficulty?

   _____

   _____

   _____

   _____

   • Why is the patient having trouble with this (these) functional subtask(s)?

   _____

   _____

   _____

   _____

   • What constraints or impairments are contributing to a particular functional limitation for that patient?

   _____

   _____

   _____

   _____

   • Of these, what constraints or impairments are removable or remediable? If so, how?

   _____

   _____

   _____

   _____

2. Patient with ataxic gait characterized by wide base, poor proximal stability at the pelvis, dysmetria, and an intention tremor affecting lower extremity limb placement and effective use of an assistive device.
   • With which functional subtasks of gait is this individual having difficulty?

   _____

   _____

   _____

   _____

   • Why is the patient having trouble with this (these) functional subtask(s)?

   _____

   _____

   _____

   _____

   • What constraints or impairments are contributing to a particular functional limitation for that patient?

   _____

   _____

   _____

   _____

   • Of these, what constraints or impairments are removable or remediable? If so, how?

_____

_____

_____

_____

3. Ten-year-old child with cerebral palsy using a reverse walker, demonstrating a crouch gait characterized by hip and knee flexion, excessive dorsiflexion, and limited pelvic movement/dissociation.
   - With which functional subtasks of gait is this individual having difficulty?

_____

_____

_____

_____

   - Why is the patient having trouble with this (these) functional subtask(s)?

_____

_____

_____

_____

   - What constraints or impairments are contributing to a particular functional limitation for that patient?

_____

_____

_____

_____

   - Of these, what constraints or impairments are removable or remediable. If so, how?

_____

_____

_____

_____

4. Eight-year-old child with cerebral palsy, demonstrating a stiff leg gait, characterized by

scissoring of the lower extremities and increased extensor muscle tone in the lower extremities, resulting in a toe-walking pattern.
   - With which functional subtasks of gait is this individual having difficulty?

_____

_____

_____

_____

   - Why is the patient having trouble with this (these) functional subtask(s)?

_____

_____

_____

_____

   - What constraints or impairments are contributing to a particular functional limitation for that patient?

_____

_____

_____

_____

   - Of these, what constraints or impairments are removable or remediable? If so, how?

_____

_____

_____

_____

5. Patient with Parkinson's disease demonstrating akinesia and bradykinesia; a flexed, stooped posture; and rigid lower extremities.
   - With which functional subtasks of gait is this individual having difficulty?

_____

_____

_____

_____

- Why is the patient having trouble with this (these) functional subtask(s)?

  _____

  _____

  _____

  _____

- What constraints or impairments are contributing to a particular functional limitation for that patient?

  _____

- Of these, what constraints or impairments are removable or remediable? If so, how?

  _____

  _____

  _____

  _____

Review Questions

1. What are the main functional tasks of the lower extremity?

2. What are the differences between the non–weight-bearing and weight-bearing functions of the lower extremity?

3. What are the common non–weight-bearing tasks of the lower extremity? What are their contributions to lower extremity function, and what are the intervention implications of this information?

4. What are the common weight-bearing tasks of the lower extremity? What are their contributions to lower extremity function, and what are the intervention implications of this information?

5. What is the importance of functional upright stance control? What are some guidelines that can be used to assist in directing intervention to establish or reestablish stance control with patients?

6. What is locomotion?

7. Why is rolling an important functional task, and how do rolling patterns change over the course of the life span?

_____

_____

_____

_____

8. What is the difference between crawling and creeping?

_____

_____

_____

_____

9. Define the following terms: kinematics, kinetics, gait cycle, stance, swing, initial contact, loading, midstance, terminal stance, preswing, initial swing, midswing, terminal swing.

_____

_____

_____

_____

10. What are the functional tasks of gait, and specifically which tasks are accomplished at each of the subphases of the gait cycle? How can an understanding of these functional tasks direct physical and occupational therapy intervention strategies?

_____

_____

_____

_____

11. What are the basic range-of-motion and muscular firing requirements at the different subphases of gait? Create a table and summarize phase by phase.

_____

_____

_____

_____

12. What are the key aspects of immature gait, and how can this knowledge affect a clinical approach to intervention for a gait disorder in a young child?

_____

_____

_____

_____

13. What are the characteristics and attributes of mature gait, and how can this knowledge affect a clinical approach to intervention for a gait disorder in an adult?

14. What are the functional effects of gait changes in the older adult, and how can these changes affect a clinical approach to intervention for a gait disorder in the older adult?

15. How does the use of an assistive or orthotic device change the functional tasks of gait?

16. What are the functional limitations consequent to the following impairments that contribute to lower extremity mobility difficulties in individuals with neurological dysfunction: weakness, interference from abnormal muscle tone, and coordination problems?

17. What effect can muscular weakness have on lower extremity function, including locomotion?

18. What effect can spasticity have on lower extremity function, including locomotion?

19. Define the terminology used to describe uncoordinated movement: ataxia, movement decomposition, dysmetria, coactivation.

_____

_____

_____

_____

20. What is the significance of musculoskeletal constraints or pain on movement, including lower extremity functional control?

_____

_____

_____

_____

21. What are some of the main functional costs of pathological gait?

_____

_____

_____

_____

22. What are some of the main pathokinematic differences in gait observed in children with cerebral palsy? How can knowledge of these factors and an understanding of developing or immature movement skills affect a clinical approach to intervention for a child with cerebral palsy?

_____

_____

_____

_____

23. What are some of the main pathokinematic characteristics of the gait of an adult with hemiplegia? Describe a functional approach to intervention for gait impairments.

_____

_____

_____

_____

24. What are the main pathokinematic characteristics of the gait of an adult with Parkinson's disease? Describe a functional approach to intervention for gait impairments.

_____

_____

_____

_____

25. What are the main pathokinematic characteristics of the gait of an individual with ataxia (child or adult)? Describe a functional approach to intervening in gait impairments.

_____

_____

_____

_____

26. What are the typical muscle tone abnormalities seen in congenital and postnatal spinal cord injury? How are they different?

_____

_____

_____

_____

Answers to Review Questions

Chapter One

1. Neuroscience is an interdisciplinary science devoted to the study of the human nervous system, evolved from several basics sciences including medicine, biology, mathematics, physics, chemistry, and psychology. Neuro-rehabilitation is the application of neuroscience to the rehabilitation of individuals with brain injury.

2. Both physical and occupational therapy are professions that are grounded in basic sciences, including neuroscience as well as the social sciences. These professions, their theories, and the subsequent frames of reference or approaches will continue to evolve as advances in all of the basic sciences and social sciences continue to emerge, develop, refine, and build.

3. Physical and occupational therapists contribute to the rehabilitation of individuals with neurological impairments by employing a wide variety of approaches to assessment and intervention, currently framed in terms of motor control as a dynamic interaction of multiple subsystems as applied to a changing human being interacting within many different environments performing a wide variety of functional tasks. In the two professions, there is an appreciation of motor control and motor learning. Occupational therapists focus on understanding the person as an *occupational* being who actively engages in meaningful and purposeful activity. Physical therapists focus on meeting an individual's functional goals by minimizing or preventing functional limitations primarily encountered within the movement system. Occupational therapy is very much grounded in the social sciences, whereas physical therapy is very much grounded in the biological and physical sciences.

4. The disablement model offers a way for clinicians to view the effect of pathological conditions on the *functioning* of body systems, on basic human performance, and on a person's ability to function in necessary, usual, and expected roles in society. This model delineates the interrelationships among pathologic conditions, impairments, functional limitations, disabilities, and handicaps or societal limitations. The role of the rehabilitation professional is to promote health through the maintenance of function, to address the functional consequences of the disease, and to prevent these consequences from initially occurring. Because physical therapists and occupational therapists can provide services to persons at risk, this model also focuses on preventive managemenal by drawing a correlation among the pathological condition, impairment, and possible functional limitations.

5. Pathophysiology is synonymous with disease, condition, or disorder; is usually consistent with the medical diagnosis; is identified primarily at the cellular level; and can be the result of many different causes, such as infection, trauma, or degenerative processes. Any single disorder may disrupt normal anatomical structures or physiological processes. For example, a diagnosis of multiple sclerosis alerts clinicians to common factors associated with the disease, but by itself the clinician is unable to understand fully the impairments and functional limitations that need to be the focus of intervention. Impairment is the typical consequence of disease or pathological processes: the loss or abnormality of physiological, psychological, or anatomical structure or function. An example of an impairment is abnormal muscle strength. Functional limitation, also termed activity limitation, is restriction of the ability to perform—at the level of the whole person— a physical action, activity, or task in an efficient, typically expected, or competent manner. An example is an inability to remove a coat from a

hanger. Disability or participation restriction is the inability to engage in age-specific and gender-specific roles in a particular social context and physical environment. It is a restricted ability to perform tasks and activities associated with self-care, home management, work, community, and leisure. An example is the inability of a child to raise his or her hand in a classroom to answer a question or to play at recess with his or her peers.

6. The *Guide to Physical Therapist Practice* standardizes terminology and delineates practice guidelines to assist therapists in physical therapy diagnosis and in the establishment of management strategies for commonly encountered diagnostic groups, included in the *Guide* as evidence-based preferred practice patterns. The *Guide to Occupational Therapy Practice* outlines the enabling process and a structure for focusing occupational therapy's domain of concern on occupational performance. It provides definitions and descriptions of terms and constructs used by the profession.

7. In both occupational and physical therapy, problem solving is seen in every conversation, every observation, and in every intervention with a patient/client. From the time a referral is received until that patient leaves the clinical environment, clinicians continually implement problem solving. Sound decision making is grounded in problem-solving skills.

8. Narrative reasoning is the type of reasoning one uses when engaged in a conversation with someone; listening carefully to the individual as he or she is led into a conversation about his or her goals, hobbies, interests, and favorite purposeful activities. An example of narrative reasoning is the information gained from a patient about his or her favorite activities and goals, which also gives the clinician insight about the individual's understanding of the nature of his or her disorder. Interactive reasoning takes place during any face-to-face encounter by gleaning information through conversation or by observation of such elements as body orientation, eye contact and eye movement, and nonverbal and verbal behavior, including voice elements. An example of interactive reasoning is lack of eye contact as signifying a person expressing difficulty confronting a conversation or situation. Pattern recognition is based on the ability to observe and interpret cues, such as recognizing that a smaller, atrophied

upper and lower extremity on one body side in a child is typically associated with hemiplegic cerebral palsy. Procedural reasoning is the type of knowledge that an experienced clinician can apply to a clinical situation because of learned professional or academic knowledge, such as the recognition of scapular instability manifested by scapular winging and ineffective upper extremity use, and anticipating the probable presence of low muscle tone or muscular weakness.

Chapter Two

1. Anatomically, the nervous system is divided into the central nervous system and the peripheral nervous system. The physiological divisions are the somatic nervous system and the autonomic nervous system.

2. A neuron is an excitable cell that receives and sends signals to other excitable cells. It is composed of a cell body, or soma, dendrites, and an axon. An axon is a single process from the neuron cell body, along which an impulse is conducted. Axons may extend for long distances, typically making contact with another neuron. Dendrites are cell processes that carry impulses toward the cell body of the neuron. Myelin is the fatty insulating substance that helps the axon conduct the message faster. Neuroglial cells are nonexcitable support cells, such as astrocytes, oligodendrocytes, Schwann's cells, and microglia. A synapse is a specialized zone where neurons communicate with each other; synapses can be axoaxonic, axosomatic, or axodendritic.

3. The nervous system sends signals by converting mechanical or chemical energy into an electrical signal, based on ionic changes and charge flow. An action potential occurs when the excitable (nerve or muscle) cell membrane undergoes a critical change from its resting state. An action potential is an all-or-none event characterized by threshold, depolarization, and hyperpolarization, followed by refractory periods. A generator potential is a local, unpropagated potential that occurs in the terminal part of the sensory nerve axon. A receptor potential is a local change in charge at the receptor end organ; when the charge is adequate, it can result in the conversion of a stimulus into electrical energy that can then be transmitted. Threshold is a critical voltage

level that must be reached before rapid depolarization of the cell membrane can occur, setting off an action potential. Stimulation of a single presynaptic excitatory neuron evokes in the postsynaptic neuron an excitatory postsynaptic potential, which is a small, local, and nontransmitted depolarization. Stimulation of a single presynaptic inhibitory neuron evokes in the postsynaptic neuron an inhibitory postsynaptic potential, which is a small, local, and nontransmitted hyperpolarization. Summation is an electrical integration of more than one postsynaptic potential, occurring simultaneously in time (temporal summation) or location (spatial summation).

4. As the human central nervous system evolved, it increased in size and complexity by adding onto more primitive brain structures. The brain is divided into three main components: brain stem, limbic system, and cerebral cortex. Clinically, it is helpful to understand the evolution of the nervous system when studying the implications of brain damage and the timing of the brain damage on activity and behavior.

5. The human nervous system starts forming when the human embryo is approximately 21 to 22 days of age and measures less than 4 mm in length. Early development is hallmarked by the formation of the neural tube. The superior end of this tube develops into the brain, and the rest of the neural tube forms the spinal cord. If there is interference in this developmental process, disabilities can occur.

6. The major anatomical divisions of the nervous system and their main functions are as follows: cerebrum—voluntary control of complex sensory and motor activities and cognitive functions such as comprehension, judgment, and attention; cerebellum—regulates balance and coordination; midbrain—houses reflex centers; pons—regulates respiratory rates; medulla—contains motor and sensory stimuli, reflex center, and control centers for heart rate and respiration; spinal cord—communicates sensory information and communicates and coordinates motor information and movement patterns.

7. The following summarizes the likely clinical picture accompanying damage to the lobes of the brain: frontal lobe—problems with motor activities and cognitive functions such as judgment, attention, mood, abstract thinking, and aggres-

sion; prefrontal lobe—problems with planning, prioritizing, and sequencing of actions into a goal-directed stream of behavior; parietal—problems with processing and giving meaning to sensory information; temporal lobe—problems with auditory discrimination and speech comprehension; occipital lobe—problems with the processing and interpretation of visual information.

8. Very generally, the right cerebral hemisphere is associated functionally with perceptual abilities, and the left cerebral hemisphere is associated functionally with language.

9. Receptors respond preferentially to one form of stimulus, such as mechanical, chemical, or thermal. The receptors convert a stimulus into a generator potential, which can then be transmitted in the central nervous system. Exteroceptors give the central nervous system information about the external world, such as through touch. Interoceptors give the central nervous system information about the viscera and inside of the body. Proprioceptors give the central nervous system information about the state and position of muscles and joints.

10. The sensory function of the muscle spindle (Figure 2–1) is provided by the location of the spindle in parallel alignment with the extrafusal or skeletal muscle fiber (EFMF). As an EFMF changes length, such as during muscle contraction or stretch, the spindle detects this length change and depolarizes an afferent sensory nerve wrapped around it, called a 1a sensory nerve (a large myelinated sensory nerve). This 1a nerve also has a critical velocity threshold, meaning that it will also only detect a length change if this change exceeds a certain rate, or velocity. If this sensory nerve depolarizes, noting a muscle stretch of a sufficient velocity, it will depolarize and send this impulse into the dorsal horn (where all sensory information enters the spinal cord), where it can connect with other neurons. It makes a direct connection (monosynaptic) to an efferent nerve, an alpha motor neuron (the anterior horn cell), which then transmits a signal back to the same EFMF, signaling the skeletal muscle to contract. The incoming sensory afferent nerve also makes an additional connection, this time through an interneuron (disynaptic) to another efferent alpha motor neuron, which then transmits a signal to the antagonist muscle, signaling that muscle to

relax. The monosynaptic component of this example is also known as the stretch reflex, a simple reflex arc mediated at the spinal cord level without cerebral influence. The motor function of the muscle spindle is conceptualized by further study of Figure 2–1. The muscle fibers at either ends of the spindle, called intrafusal muscle fibers (IFMFs), are innervated by gamma efferent nerves, whose cell bodies are located in the ventral, or anterior, horn of the spinal cord. These gamma cells, however, receive synaptic connections and influences from throughout the human nervous system, such as the cortex, cerebellum, and brain stem. This constant volley of regulatory input onto the IFMFs of the muscle spindle through the collective input onto the gamma nerves sets up a constant resting state of readiness so that skeletal muscle is literally on a steady state of alert or arousal for the task demands to be placed on it. This constant state of readiness is called muscle tone; further clarified, it is normal muscle tone when the inputs onto this system are absent of pathological conditions. The contribution of the muscle spindle is only one piece of the puzzle contributing to the phenomenon called muscle tone. The spindles, however, play a crucial role by providing ongoing feedback to the nervous system about the changing conditions of muscle length.

11. Meninges are inside the vertebral column and the cranium. They encase the nervous system, offering protection from infection and contusion. Cerebrospinal fluid is formed within the ventricles in the brain and is the cushion for the nervous system, offering support, transportation of nutrients, and removal of metabolic wastes.

12. The main arteries of cerebral circulation are the carotid arteries, anterior cerebral artery, middle cerebral artery, posterior cerebral artery, and the vertebral arteries. The Circle of Willis is the name of the circular arrangement of cerebral blood vessels, another method whereby the central nervous system preserves function in the face of injury or pathological process.

13. Anterior cerebral artery pathology often produces contralateral weakness and sensory loss primarily in the lower extremity, aphasia, memory and behavioral deficits, and incontinence. Middle cerebral artery pathology often produces contralateral weakness and sensory loss in the face and upper extremity, with less involvement in the lower extremity. Posterior cerebral artery pathology often produces contralateral sensory loss, thalamic pain syndrome, homonymous hemianopsia, visual agnosia, and cortical blindness. Vertebrobasilar cerebral artery pathology often produces cranial nerve involvement, difficulty swallowing, and dysarthria.

14. Focal lesions are limited to a single location. An example of this type of lesion is stroke, where the blood supply is occluded, and a specific area of the brain loses its blood supply. In this situation, it is entirely possible to ascribe most of a patient's symptoms to a loss of function in that specific area of the brain. Multifocal lesions are limited to several, nonsymmetrical locations. An example of this type of lesion is multiple sclerosis, in which lesions develop over time in different locations. The signs and symptoms of this patient are multiple, with the presentation of new signs or symptoms perhaps indicative of spread or progression of the disease. Diffuse lesions affect bilaterally symmetrical structures but not crossing midline as a single lesion. Diffuse dysfunction of the nervous system can be produced by a number of toxins or metabolic disturbances, frequently alerting the examiner to look for a systemic disorder giving rise to such a multitude of signs.

15. Weakness is an inability to generate normal levels of muscular force. Depending on the extent of the lesion, weakness in the patient with a cerebral cortex lesion can vary in severity from total loss of muscle activity to minimal impairment. Muscle tone is determined by the level of excitability of the entire pool of motor neurons controlling a muscle, the intrinsic stiffness of the muscle itself, the absence of neuropathology, and the level of sensitivity of many different reflexes. Abnormal muscle tone can be characterized as hypotonia, flaccidity, spasticity, or rigidity. Flaccidity is the complete loss of muscle tone. In patients who experience flaccidity, tendon reflexes are absent, and the muscle feels very floppy. Hypotonia is a reduction in muscle stiffness, characterized by low muscle tone, weak proximal muscle control, poor muscular co-contraction, and limited stability. Spasticity is a form of abnormally high muscle tone and can limit a patient's ability to move quickly. Usually, voluntary active muscle control is severely weakened. Rigidity is a form of abnormally high muscle tone characterized by heightened resistance to passive movement, predominant in the flexor muscles of the trunk and limbs. Dystonia is a syndrome characterized by sustained muscle

contractions, frequently causing abnormal postures, twisting or writhing movements, and repetitive abnormal postures. Tremor is a rhythmical, involuntary, oscillatory movement of a body part. Uncoordinated movement may be displayed through the manifestation of abnormal synergies, inappropriate coactivation patterns, and timing problems.

16. Vicarious function theory states that the undamaged central nervous system regions have latent capabilities that can respond to or control actions originally handled by the damaged areas. Equipotentiality states that various parts of the nervous system can mediate the same motor functions. Functional reorganization theory suggests that a neural system can alter its function depending on the need and secondary to damage to related areas. The theory of substitution proposes that a motor behavior can be performed by a mechanism different than that which originally controlled the behavior.

17. There are several differences between developmental and adult neuroplasticity. The growth of adult axons is very restricted later in life. Dendrite formation occurs throughout life but not to the extent that it occurs during early development. The plasticity that is associated with early development is heavily reliant on structural changes, such as cell growth, migration, and the formation of axons, dendrites, and synapses. The plastic changes available to adults are generally considered due not to actual structural change but to changes in synaptic strength and efficiency.

Chapter Three

1. Both physical and occupational therapy are professions that are grounded in basic sciences, including neuroscience as well as the social sciences. These professions, their theories, and the subsequent frames of reference, intervention approaches, and practice models will continue to evolve as advances in all of the basic sciences and social sciences continue to emerge, develop, refine, and build. The practice arena and depth of practice should grow together with growth in the body of knowledge.

2. Understanding the science of movement control evolved from a reflex model to a hierarchical or neuromaturational model to, most recently, a motor control model grounded in a systems

approach and a dynamic action systems model. The reflex model first suggested that movement was the result of a summation of sensory input to the central nervous system and that the nervous system controlled the execution of movement based on the sensory feedback received. The hierarchical model suggested that movements were controlled in a top-down fashion, originating from the central nervous system. These models have shifted to a systems model that recognizes the dynamic nature of movement and the adaptable contributions of many subsystems to the integration of human movement.

3. The dynamic systems approach views movement as emerging from the cooperation of many subsystems in a task-specific context. The many systems then self-organize to produce movement and do not depend on prior instruction embodied in one hierarchically important subsystem. Each component is perceived as necessary but insufficient, by itself, to explain movement.

4. The systems approach allows the practitioner to view the central nervous system as subservient to functional purpose, in which structures may contribute to more than one function and thereby be a part of more than one system.

5. The application of a systems approach consists of examining the patient/client in a holistic manner, whereby the status of every subsystem within the individual may affect the movement outcome. The movement that the clinician observes as demonstrated by the patient represents the sum of the interactions of all these contributing systems.

6. The systems involved are dynamic in nature due to the fact that the subsystems change over time. Each subsystem continually adapts to change. Every subsystem has its own unique developmental timeline. Movement production, therefore, at any given moment is the best product created from the contributory inputs of *all* interacting systems in *that* environment and responding to *that* specific movement instance.

7. The concept of life-span development encompasses all developmental changes—those generally associated with childhood and adolescence as well as the changes that take place with aging. Early development typically applies to beginning prenatal growth and organization of each system. Maturation occurs during infancy and

childhood and continues through adolescence. During maturation the qualitative changes enable an individual to progress to a higher level of functioning. Maturity is associated with adulthood. It implies a period of relative stability, with most changes driven by individual responses to environmental or task demands. Aging refers to the changes in physical, sensory, and psychosocial performance that occur to some extent in all elderly persons over time.

8. From conception through the second year of life, the human nervous system is in a tremendous wave of development and change. The main processes guiding these early changes are cell migration and differentiation, axonal growth, dendritic formation, neurotransmitter synthesis, and the formation of synapses. These dramatic changes that occur in the developing brain do not occur again in later life. In early development, the central nervous system actually overgrows. Regressive processes such as cell death and the retraction of some projections, which follow subsequent to this initial overgrowth, are an equally important part of early development. By birth, the human newborn has the full complement of neurons; all have migrated to their final destination point. From 8 weeks gestation through age 3 years, myelination is the main nervous system task. For example, the acquisition of myelin sheaths by the spinal nerves and roots by the 10th week of life is associated with the beginning of the first reflex motor activities, such as sucking and fetal kicking. Myelination occurs first in those areas of the nervous system that will be used first, laid down in the areas of the brain stem and cranial nerves involved in reflexive sucking and swallowing. Myelin formation in the central nervous system begins at the sixth month of gestation, continuing into adulthood.

9. Recovery or even maintenance of a function appears to depend on the stage of development of the damaged pathway and also on the stage of development of the undamaged pathways. It is well accepted that critical periods exist whereby damage to various parts of the central nervous system will have different behavioral effects depending on whether the damage occurs prior to or after this critical period. Critical periods are times when axons are competing for synaptic sites and pathways are organizing. The concept of critical periods has important clinical implications. For example, if input from one area or sensory receptor is dysfunctional during the crit-

ical period for that region or structure, the axons are at a disadvantage as they compete for synaptic space. Permanent neural change will result. Various central nervous system structures have different critical periods with different durations.

10. Early development of the central nervous system is hallmarked by system overgrowth, axon and dendritic formation/growth, synapse formation, cell migration, regional differentiation, and some myelination. Maturation is characterized by increased myelination, especially of the cerebral hemispheres and corticospinal tract, neuronal growth and maturation, and increased complexity of neuronal processes. Increased myelination of the association areas, synaptic remodeling, and the beginning signs of decline in nerve conduction velocities and brain weight hallmark maturity. Aging is characterized by a decrease in number of neurons and neuronal shrinkage and a decrease in frontal and temporal lobe volume and cerebellar size, although dendrites continue to grow even into old age. Knowledge of all these changes can increase the breadth and depth of a clinician's understanding in working with clients of all ages.

11. The somatosensory system includes all those structures involved in the reception of signals (receptors), the dorsal root of the spinal cord, the thalamus, the sensory cortex (predominately parietal), and the afferent tracts, which carry this information.

12. The somatosensory system includes all those structures involved from the reception of signals from the periphery to the integration and interpretation of those signals relative to all the simultaneous incoming information. At best, somatosensory information can be modulated at every level, contributing to a smooth execution of movement most appropriate for the task within the environmental context. Somatosensory inputs provide crucial information to the central nervous system for effective postural control and movement execution. Sensation is paired with movement in the form of reflexes. Sensation is also used as feedback to refine movement and as a stimulus for postural responses. Somatosensation contributes to the production of smooth, purposeful movement.

13. Somatosensory pathways are the earliest to develop and are almost completely myelinated at birth. Conduction velocities increase, myelination increases, and synapses increase in

efficiency during maturation. With age, sensation is still used to reinforce or refine new movements, but the speed of processing sensory information declines. With age, there is a decrease in the numbers of several types of sensory neurons, a decline in functioning of the remaining sensory neurons, and actual structural and physiological changes within the central nervous system. Because of changes in the senses, clinicians need to focus on safety issues, and the therapist or assistant may need to use additional cues for the older adult. Knowledge of all these changes can increase the breadth and depth of a clinician's understanding in working with clients of all ages.

14. The visual system is divided into a peripheral portion and the central visual pathway. The peripheral structures include the eye, its photoreceptors, and several different cells that either respond to stimuli or relay visual information. The visual system allows an individual to identify objects in space and determine their movement. It also supplies information about where the body is in space, about the relation of one body part to another, and the motion of one's own body. This system plays a vital role in posture control, locomotion, balance, and hand function.

15. The central visual pathways and the eye itself develop very early in development. Maturation and adulthood are hallmarked by increased acuity, increased maturation, and processing. During the aging process, less light is transmitted to the retina; therefore, the visual threshold increases with age, requiring more light to see an object. Pupil sizes decrease with age, allowing less light into the eye. There is a decrease in the ability to adapt from dark to light environments. Older adults also demonstrate narrower peripheral vision. Depth perception and contrast sensitivity decrease sharply between the ages of 60 and 75 years. Older adults also have a decline in central processing. During therapy, an older adult may need more sensory, verbal, or physical cues in order to execute tasks and maintain successful independence. Clinicians may observe the tendency for older adults to require additional support, such as a handrail. Knowledge of all these changes can increase the breadth and depth of a clinician's understanding in working with clients of all ages.

16. The vestibular system originates in each ear and projects directly into the brain, divides, and extends as far superiorly as the cerebral cortex and as far caudally as the spinal cord. The system is divided into a peripheral and central component. The vestibular system signals changes in head position or motion referenced by the pull of gravity. This system provides information about position and coordinated postural movements. It provides information concerning center of gravity, rotation, and acceleration.

17. The vestibular system is completely myelinated at birth but continuing maturation and integration occur throughout maturation. Disordered balance in the elderly is probably due to a manifestation of deterioration in central vestibular integrative functions. Vestibular problems cause dizziness and unsteadiness when an individual is in an environment with conflicting or unfamiliar visual and somatosensory inputs. Clinicians need to be aware that a decline in the vestibular system can cause dizziness and vertigo in older adults. Falls are also more common in the elderly population, possibly due to a less reliable vestibular system. Knowledge of all these changes can increase the breadth and depth of a clinician's understanding in working with clients of all ages.

18. The motor cortex, including the primary motor cortex, the supplementary motor area, and the premotor cortex, all in the frontal lobe, interacts with sensory processing areas in the parietal lobe and with basal ganglia and cerebellar areas to identify where an individual wants to move, to plan the movement, and to execute the movement.

19. The musculoskeletal system forms, organizes, and grows during maturation and into maturity. During the aging process, the individual will experience a decrease in muscular strength and loss of both types of muscle fibers, and the skeletal system becomes more compromised. Muscular wasting and changes in flexibility are also associated with the aging process. Knowledge of all these changes can increase the breadth and depth of a clinician's understanding in working with clients of all ages.

Chapter Four

1. Development can be thought of as a change in form and function where form and function are intertwined. Growth refers to an increase in size

and weight, changes in the physical dimensions of the body. Maturation is the increase in complexity within body systems, allowing more sophisticated functioning. Adaptation occurs secondary to stimuli placed upon the system, such as the modeling that occurs within bone secondary to muscle pull.

2. Motor development is the process of change in motor behavior that is related to the age of the individual. Motor development is a life-span event: age-related change in motor behavior is an ongoing, lifelong phenomenon hallmarked by all the processes and factors that contribute to these age-related changes.

3. Sensitive periods suggest that appropriate intervention during a specific period tends to facilitate more positive forms of development than if the same intervention occurs at another time.

4. Resiliency means that development is an individual, dynamic process that can adapt and modify in response to both intrinsic and extrinsic variables as it unfolds.

5. Piaget developed a theory of intelligence in which cognitive development is divided into four stages: sensorimotor, preoperational, concrete operational, and formal operations. Piaget's theory focuses on how important problem-solving activities within the intervention setting are to assist in the cognitive and motivational aspects of facilitating motor development. The theory reminds clinicians that movement does not occur spontaneously or without purpose. When training or retraining movement, clinicians should actively engage the mover in problem solving.

6. Erikson's theory describes the developmental stages that a person goes through to establish personality. Clinicians working with individuals at different times of the life span should be sensitive to what primary developmental tasks are the main focuses at that age stage.

7. Neuromaturational theory viewed development as occurring along a sequence of stages, with reflexes being the basic building blocks of movement. Clinicians are urged not to disregard valuable assessments and intervention insights and tools that emerged from these theorists. These theories resulted in the development of important tests of motor milestones and have had a profound influence in the diagnosis of developmental delay.

8. The dynamic systems theory provides a more holistic approach to the understanding of human motor development. This theory suggests that control of movement is the result of many contributing subsystems working together dynamically. The model implies that no one factor has greater influence than the others. For clinicians using this theory, it is important to explore the movement possibilities and flexible selection of the most appropriate movement synergy or preferred pattern for accomplishing goal-directed behavior.

9. The term cephalocaudal is used to describe development that proceeds in a general direction from head to foot. Developmental change is also generally observed as proceeding in a proximal to distal direction, in reference to the midline of the body; for example, a person will have difficulty using a computer if the individual's trunk is not stabilized. Gross movement is a large, undefined, or mass movement; for example, an infant swiping at a large object with the entire upper extremity. Fine movement is a more refined, precise movement; for example, an infant picking up tiny objects with his or her fingers. The descriptors undifferentiated and specific describe how the infant or adult may first move the entire body in response to a stimulus before a more specific response emerges. In infancy, this is illustrated by rolling: the infant rolls in a mass, log-like fashion in which the entire body moves as a unit before a more specific dissociated response emerges.

10. Physiological flexion is used to describe the predominantly flexed posture of a full-term newborn infant. Antigravity extension is the voluntary, active movement, first of the neck and then of the trunk, against the force of gravity; for example, first evident in prone with the head lifting and then extension of the trunk. Antigravity flexion develops as the baby combats the force of gravity first in the supine and sidelying positions, evident by head lifting, foot play in supine, beginning bridging, and successful voluntary movement out of supine. Mobility is the movement function, in which moving is the main task goal; for example, an infant's random movements of arms and legs. Stability is the movement function in which the holding of a posture is the main task goal; for example, an infant

being able to hold itself up using the elbows in a prone position. Asymmetry evolves to symmetry and then to controlled asymmetry. An infant may demonstrate early movement characterized by asymmetry: not having the two sides of the body performing the same movement. More mature movement patterns may be evidenced by more symmetrical movements, which is the idea that what one side of the body does is what the other side does. Controlled asymmetry is evidenced by movement whereby the extremities are dissociated from each other and from the trunk and head, evidenced by mature locomotion and upper extremity use. Weight-bearing experiences assist in the development of stability. Adequate weight-bearing is made possible through stability around the proximal girdle, the scapula/shoulder for the upper extremity, and the pelvis for the lower extremity. In order to move with control, weight shifting must occur. Weight shifting occurs as one body part stabilizes simultaneously with the other body part being unweighted enough to move. Weight bearing and weight shifting are used throughout changes in position and posture. Rotation can be demonstrated because of a balanced control of both flexors and extensors and dissociation between body segments. Rotation through the trunk allows for such milestones as moving to sitting from prone, rotating within sitting, creeping, reaching on all fours, and moving to stance through half kneel and locomotion. Dissociation is the ability to move one body part or segment without an associated movement of another body part or segment as seen in the breaking up of mass movement patterns, characterized by the ability to separate movement in one body part from associated movement in another. Examples of dissociation include the dissociation of the shoulders from the trunk and the hips from the pelvis as seen in mature rolling, dissociation of the lower extremities from each other during gait, and dissociation of the upper extremities from the trunk during ball playing and reciprocal arm swinging during gait. Rotation and fluid dissociation also permit self-help skills such as independent dressing.

11. The movement development sequence is based on building upon previously attained skills but not as rigid building blocks in a fixed order. Each movement as it emerges and is practiced is slightly different from what was learned before. The mover participates in and influences the emergence, practice, and mastery of his or her own movement skills. Developmental change occurs because of active problem solving. "Sequence" is a troublesome term because it may be construed as meaning rigid and fixed, which developmental change is not.

12. Motor milestones assist the rehabilitation clinician because they offer landmarks for recognizing the key skills that are typically mastered as increased independence and movement sophistication emerge. These milestones are also helpful to chart progress toward development of skill.

13. Some of the main gross milestones are as follows: newborn—rolls partly to side, in prone turns head to side, and reflexive standing and stepping; 2 months—spontaneous rolling sidelying to supine, partial or full head lag, and lifts head in prone to 45 degrees; 3 to 5 months—prone prop onto forearms, plays with feet in supine, will stand with support, and head control; 6 months—belly crawling, rolls supine to prone, and plays in sidelying; 7 to 9 months—pivots in sitting, cruising, and assumes quadruped and rocks; 10 to 12 months—pulls to stand through half kneel, walks with one or two hands held; 18 months—rises to stand without pulling up, squats to pick up objects, and walks up stairs nonreciprocally; 2 to 3 years—rides tricycle, begins to run, and climbs playground equipment; 4 to 6 years—begins to skip, kicks and bounces large ball, and hops a few feet; 6 to 10 years—mastery of adult forms of running and jumping, hops and skips skillfully, and postural control is adult-like. Adolescence is characterized by the development of specialized movement skills such as dodging, balancing, and success in sports requiring volleying and trapping.

14. Some of the fine motor milestones are as follows: newborn—grasp reflex and random upper extremity movements in supine; 2 months—palmar grasp, recognizes hands, and primitive reaching behaviors; 3 to 5 months—grasps and releases toys, primitive squeezing (raking), and fingers to mouth; 6 months—voluntary palmar grasp, finger feeds, and attempts at holding cup and spoon; 7 to 9 months—radial palmar grasp, transfers objects from hand to hand, and develops active forearm supination; 10 to 12 months—three-jaw chuck, can stack two cubes, and increased independence in feeding and undressing; 18 months—hand preference begins to

emerge, controlled grasp and release, and turns container over to empty contents; 2 to 3 years— pencil or crayon held by finger and thumb, turns knob, and unscrews jars; 4 to 6 years—printing skills and skilled hand use to manipulate utensils; 6 to 10 years—handwriting and keyboarding skills, increased coordination with manipulating small objects, and throws and catches with increased mastery. Adolescence is hallmarked by increased movement mastery such as skillful ball playing due to increased eye-hand coordination and increased dexterity in tasks.

15. A reflex is a largely automatic, somewhat stereotypical, consistent, and predictable motor response to a specific stimulus, usually sensory. It is a preferred movement pattern at specific times. An example is a stepping reflex or the asymmetrical tonic neck reflex. A righting reaction is a postural response of the head or trunk, elicited secondary to displacement or movement, ensuring the realignment of the head and trunk with each other or with regard to an outside stimulus. Examples include head and trunk righting. Equilibrium reactions adjust for a change in the body's orientation in space, composed of righting responses of the head and trunk and protective extension responses of the extremities. Equilibrium reactions are present in all positions, such as sitting and standing. Protective extension is the extension motion of the upper or lower extremities toward the supporting surface, elicited in preparation for catching oneself from a fall. Associated reactions are movements of a body part that occur involuntarily in accompaniment to another movement, such as biting one's tongue during concentrated work or curling one's toes when balance is challenged.

16. Functional movements are the movement patterns that are used for or adapted to a function or a group of similar functions.

17. The main functional movement components required for successful postural control of the head and trunk are head and trunk movements in anterior, posterior, and lateral directions. The muscles of the neck and trunk must be able to work isometrically, concentrically, and eccentrically.

18. The main functional movement components required for successful upper extremity control are either those required for movement in space or for weight-bearing movements. The key func-

tional components are the ability to reach forward, reach into abduction away from the body, reach backward, reach away from the midline, reach across midline, and the ability to position the elbow and hand.

19. The main functional movement components required for successful lower extremity control are the ability to support body weight on both legs, to transfer weight from one leg to the other, to bear weight on one leg and then move the other leg, and to constantly adapt to movements of the trunk and upper extremities.

20. The first year of life serves as a model demonstrating the eventual development of postural control and of extremity control evidenced by increasing mastery over movement within the environment. See text for details.

21. Postural control and control of the extremities go through many age-related changes, as each contributing subsystem develops uniquely. See text for details.

22. During the aging process, postural sway in standing increases, and movement patterns again become increasingly asymmetrical. Hand strength, performance time, and the frequency with which varying prehension patterns are used are affected by age. Older adults show decreased reaction time, and tactile sensation is decreased. Gait characteristics common to older adults include a wider base of support, decreased reciprocal arm swing, and slower cadence. Stride length decreases, and time in double support increases.

Chapter Five

1. Learning is defined as a relatively permanent change in the capability for responding, which occurs as a result of practice or experience. Training occurs when the performer is provided with solutions to problems. Performance is defined as a temporary change in behavior readily observable during practice sessions.

2. Motor control is the study of the nature and cause of movement, focusing on the control and coordination of the movement and posture. Motor control emerges from an interaction between the individual, the task, and the environment. Motor learning is concerned with how motor skills are acquired. The factors that affect motor learning are environmental conditions,

cognitive processes, and movement organization. Therapists and assistants provide feedback, opportunities to practice, and encouragement to patients in order to affect that individual's motor learning.

3. Learning and memory involve a change in the internal structure of neurons and an increase in the number of synapses. They involve both parallel and hierarchical processing within the central nervous system, and multiple parallel information channels are used.

4. Habituation involves a decrease in a behavior due to repeated exposure to a nonpainful stimulus (example: procedures used to decrease tactile defensiveness). Sensitization involves an increased responsiveness to a threatening or noxious stimulus (example: stimulating activities used to arouse a comatose patient). Perceptual learning involves the formation of sensory memories, which can serve as a spontaneous rehearsal mechanism for that action or occurrence (example: visual demonstration of a new skill to a patient).

5. Classical conditioning involves learning to pair stimuli in a process whereby an initially weak stimulus becomes highly effective in producing a response when it is associated with another stronger stimulus (example: babies appearing to fear doctors or nurses in white coats and the medical setting because these characteristics are associated with pain). Operant conditioning involves trial-and-error learning whereby the learner associates a certain response, among many that have been made, with a consequence (example: patient gains skills, the patient progresses along a continuum of levels of assistance, and the new behavior is shaped by the therapist or assistant as the learner acquires new skills). Procedural learning is the process whereby a task is learned by forming movement habits (example: patient practices safe and effective transfers in a variety of settings and contexts). Declarative learning results in knowledge that can be continuously recalled and thus requires processes such as awareness and attention (example: the clinician verbally explains a procedure to a patient and allows the patient to practice the movement mentally before or between the practice sessions).

6. Adam's closed-loop theory is credited with introducing the importance of practice and the value of retraining in motor reeducation.

Schmidt's schema theory suggests that a motor program is a generalized prestructured plan that can be modified according to the specific task demands, supporting the concept that practicing a variety of movement outcomes improves learning through the development of expanded rules or schema. Ecological theory emphasizes the dynamic nature of movement exploration and the problem solving actively engaged in while learning a task within specific constraints and in a variable environment.

7. The environment should provide the opportunity for active participation from the learner (patient) so that the setting is a viable learning environment. Understand the patient's needs. Environmental stressors such as bright lights and noise should be minimized. Tasks should be practiced in environments in which they naturally occur.

8. Arousal refers to the overall level of alertness or excitement of the cerebral cortex. High arousal is associated with high energy or excitement, and low arousal is associated with sleep or feelings of drowsiness. Attention is the capacity of the brain to process information from the environment or retrieve information from long-term memory. Attention includes the patient's ability to be aware of and respond to a stimulus, to focus on the desired information and ignore irrelevant information, to shift the focus to other information if necessary, and to sustain the focus. Motivation is the internal state that tends to direct or energize a system toward the goal, described as a force that leads to task engagement or sustained involvement in a task.

9. Instructions can be used for motivational purposes but also for clarity of conveying the information to the learner about the task. Instructions can focus the patient's attention on different levels of information about the task. Guidance is most effective during the early phases of learning (skill acquisition). Clinicians are reminded that overuse of guidance will promote dependency and can actually interfere with motor learning.

10. Feedback refers to the use of sensory information for the control of action in the process of skill acquisition. Intrinsic feedback (from within the learner) and extrinsic feedback (from an outside source) are the types of feedback that are used in clinical practice. The type of feedback employed should be patient-specific, matching

the abilities of the learner and enhancing the ability of that unique individual to learn. As learning increases, feedback should be faded or decreased in both frequency and quantity.

11. Practice is the continuing and repetitive effort to become proficient in a skill. Physical practice is a type of practice that allows the learner to gain direct experience, crucial for the shaping of a motor program. Mental practice is the cognitive rehearsal of a motor task without any overt movement. Practice can be organized around the repetition of one task repeatedly, as in constant practice, or several variations of the same or similar tasks can be performed. Practice can also be organized by manipulating the frequency and duration of rest periods. Practice order (the sequence in which the tasks are practiced) is the final organization consideration.

12. The patient in the cognitive stage of learning needs information about the goal of the action and some idea of how the goal is to be accomplished. The patient is facing the task of *what* to do, such as where to place the hands before attempting a sit-to-stand transfer. Some of the clinical strategies useful during the cognitive stage are to closely structure the environment, reduce stimuli, and minimize stress. Organize practice by breaking down tasks into parts, using manual guidance to assist if appropriate. Lastly, select the appropriate use of feedback, perhaps frequently initially and reducing later as learning proceeds.

13. The patient in the associative stage of learning associates the movement attempts and the feedback received with the outcome. Performance improves, and errors are diminished over time. Clinicians should continue to structure the environment but progress to a more open one, stressing the importance of function and task meaningfulness. Organize the practice to focus on a more variable practice order in an attempt to increase retention. Lastly, select the appropriate use of feedback, emphasizing proprioceptive awareness and the ability of the patient to self-assess.

14. During the autonomous stage of learning, a shift is made to performance becoming more automatic. Movements are largely error-free, with little interference from environmental distractions. The clinician should open and vary the environment, preparing the patient for multiple settings. Vary the practice, stressing consistency of performance in variable environments with some task variation. Provide only occasional feedback, and encourage the learner to develop increased self-evaluation skills.

15. The Gentile model emphasizes the uniqueness of the learner and the learner's goal. The learner needs to develop an understanding of the task and the requirement of the movement. Regulatory conditions are characteristics of the performance environment that influence the characteristics of the movement used to perform the skill. Nonregulatory conditions are characteristics of the performance environment that are irrelevant and do not influence the movement characteristics of the skill. Open skills are skills that require diversification of the basic movement pattern acquired during the first stage of learning so that the learner is required to adapt to continuously changing regulatory conditions. Closed skills are skills that require fixation, meaning that the learner works toward developing the capability to perform the pattern automatically and efficiently. Explicit learning is a process that develops an initial mapping between the performer's body and environmental conditions, requiring active processing of information and effort during practice. Implicit learning occurs with repeated practice as the learner attempts to anticipate more precisely what is needed in order to be more efficient.

16. Learning in a natural environment facilitates skill acquisition because of familiarity, skill transfer, and retention. Purpose and occupational embeddedness increase the meaningfulness of the task to the learner. Goal-directed activity provides for meaningfulness and purpose. All of these can dramatically increase learning.

17. During childhood, play is a mechanism for an elaboration on experience, for exploration, for social development, for the development of coordination skills, and for further cognitive processing. Therapy is a teaching and learning experience. Children of different ages or levels of experience or ability have different developmental tasks, skills, and strategies for play.

18. Adults tend to have a problem-solving orientation to learning. Real-life situations and problems are the main motivator for an adult learner. Clinicians should understand that adult learning is enhanced by repetition, tasks that are more meaningful are more fully and easily learned, and environmental factors affect learning.

19. Over the life span of an individual, psychomotor skills decline, and pain and poor physical health can affect performance. A person's ability to learn a new task depends on intelligence, learning skills acquired over the years, and flexibility of learning style as well as noncognitive factors. When working with the older adult, clinicians should try to reduce the potential for distraction in an attempt to increase concentration. Allow the individual to set the learning pace. Older adults may need more time to integrate new learning and to rehearse the learning before it becomes assimilated into memory.

20. Therapists and assistants can maximize optimal learning opportunities for individuals with mental retardation and other cognitive impairments by being respectful of the nature of the person's capabilities and limitations. Attainment of fundamental movement skills is typically delayed, so additional practice time should be expected. Some patients with mental retardation may not be able to achieve a level of skillful mastery, but individual levels of functional performance should be welcomed.

21. Individuals with brain injuries may experience memory loss, and memory is needed to learn new skills. The ability to process information and subsequent learning will likely change over the first week, during the acute stage of a brain injury. With a cerebrovascular accident, deficits can occur in perception, communication, and cognition. All of these deficits may affect the ability of the patient to attend, learn, and retain information. Parkinson's disease produces difficulty with initiation, absence, or reduction in the amount of movement, difficulty stopping movement especially once momentum has taken over, and difficulty monitoring posture and making postural adjustments. All of these factors may influence learning. See the text for details.

Chapter Six

1. A theoretical model is developed to guide a particular assessment and intervention approach or frame of reference. New practical ideas are born from theoretical advances, and clinical inquiry prompts theoretical advances. Theoretical models and clinical intervention approaches reinforce each other, prompting continual inquiry, insight, and change in the practice arena.

2. The reflex theory proposed that movement is peripherally driven, wherein the sensory system literally drives motor output. Once a stimulus is provided, a response is thought to be produced throughout the nervous system, resulting in movement. This model suggested that sensory input regulated motor output. The hierarchical model was based on the idea that there are central control mechanisms that separate reflex from voluntary control patterns. The control of movement was thought to be organized hierarchically, with the spinal cord providing reflex motor patterns, the brain stem providing static or tonic reflex control and integration, and the cerebral cortex superseding all lower structures with voluntary control mechanisms. The contributions from these early theories are still of value, as now assimilated into a much broader perspective. Contemporary motor theory has a more dynamic view of the role of automatic movements (including reflexes) and their role in motor control. We now appreciate that whereas reflexes may provide a general framework or bias for movement, they do not solely address the dynamic and adaptive nature of early infant motor behavior. Current concepts recognize the fact that each level of the nervous system can act on other levels, depending on the task. Reflexive patterns of movement are not considered to be the sole determinant of motor control, but they are one of many processes important to the generation and control of movement.

3. The guiding principles of the dynamic system approach are as follows. Individuals with movement difficulties caused by neurological dysfunction are faced with constraints to movement, and there are many sources of constraints to action, some within the environment, the individual, or the task itself. Individuals with neurological disorders may present with a problem with the appropriate number of degrees of freedom necessary for unimpaired task execution. Therapeutic intervention strategies are offered by the therapist or assistant as actions that interact with the boundary conditions already present within the individual, the environment, or the attempted task. The clinician is a *change agent* working with the patient/client to generate movement, and the clinician can physically manipulate the environment, provide augmented information, or physically manipulate the individual in order to optimize the movement outcome.

4. The sensorimotor approach, emerging out of the

reflex and hierarchical models, was first proposed for intervention with individuals with a neurological impairment. The manual facilitation and inhibition techniques were the common theme in this early approach. Today's clinicians can still glean some useful concepts from these approaches, underscoring the power of a clinician's hands to alter, encourage, coax, or help to refine a patient's attempt at movement. The text offers a thorough, contemporary review of these approaches and lists in table form a practical application of these manual techniques as integrated into a holistic dynamic approach to intervention.

5. The key intervention concepts central to the proprioceptive neuromuscular facilitation are as follows. During the acquisition of functional motor skills, many key patterns of movement are recognizable; the therapist or assistant encourages the individual to focus on the goal of movement. Intervention begins with assessment of the individual's functional performance, and facilitation techniques are methods used to assist individuals in attaining their own functional movement goals. See Table 6–2 in the text or Table 6–1 in this workbook for details and clinical suggestions.

6. Intervention using the neurodevelopmental approach proposes that motor skills develop from an interaction among many systems, including the sensory systems, and that postural control and alignment provide a foundation for complex functional skill development. Intervention targets proximal and distal control, active movement, and graded facilitation through judicious use of positioning, handling, and sensory input. Intervention emphasizes consistency of handling, maximization of the therapist's sensory feedback through manual contacts, participation of the mover, creation of a motivating environment, use of ongoing assessment, incorporation of movement into functional activities, and use of preventive strategies such as adaptive equipment and orthotic devices. Neurodevelopmental theory and motor learning theory are highly complementary. See the text for details, including Table 6–3, which summarizes some intervention suggestions.

7. Although the actual approach to treatment is considered outdated and inappropriate today, Brunnstrom is credited with two main contributions that are still valuable: a description of the stereotypical synergy patterns and the recovery

stages of patients seen following a cerebrovascular accident. Brunnstrom carefully observed thousands of stroke survivors, and she meticulously recorded her observations of their movement patterns in the weeks and months following the strokes. Repeated use of synergies, which makes isolated motor control more difficult, is viewed now as inappropriate and undesirable. However, it is important that clinicians recognize the presence of a synergy if it dominates movement and interferes with voluntary movement attempts. An appreciation of this detailed observational knowledge provided by Brunnstrom is extremely helpful to clinicians and patients today. Those observations on movement highlight the importance of the current emphasis on working toward the goal of voluntary functional control and of the functional limitations experienced by patients as they work toward recovery. Brunnstrom's description of the stages of recovery is summarized as follows. The initial flaccid stage is characterized by an absence of muscular contraction. Beginning spasticity then becomes evident. Limited voluntary movement out of the synergy pattern hallmarks spasticity. Spasticity then begins to decline, and voluntary control begins to improve. Spasticity continues to decrease, and voluntary control improves. Minimal spasticity remains, and the patient begins to have good voluntary control. Full recovery is evidenced by a return to normal muscle tone and full voluntary control. The rate and recovery outcome is highly individualized. The synergy patterns are described in the text and depicted in Figure 6–7 of the text.

8. The incorporation of sensory stimulation techniques into remediation approaches is based largely on the original work of Margaret Rood. Sensory stimuli such as approximation or resistance were used to assist in the development of control in a stability activity, such as holding in a sitting position. Sensory stimuli, such as tapping and quick tactile inputs, were used to facilitate a mobility response, such as initiating a movement or activating a muscular response. Although this neurophysiology is outdated, the concept of viewing movement development as requiring the key component aspects of mobility, stability, and combinations of mobility and stability is still insightful, offering valuable clinical guideposts.

9. The three main concepts of the sensory integration frame of reference are as follows. Learning is dependent on the ability to take in and process

sensation from movement and the environment and use it to plan and organize behavior. Individuals who have a decreased ability to process sensation may also have difficulty producing appropriate actions and, in turn, may interfere with learning and behavior; enhanced sensation improves the ability to process sensation, thereby enhancing learning behavior. During intervention, controlled sensory input may be used to help individuals experience sensation, explore the environment, and process the sensations within a movement or learning task.

10. Sensorimotor techniques can still be useful as part of an integrated holistic approach to intervention. Key application concepts from the neurofacilitation/sensorimotor approaches still influence the way clinicians examine and intervene with patients who have central nervous system pathology. In current approaches, there is greater emphasis on explicitly training function and less emphasis on retraining for "normal" patterns of movement. There is more consideration of motor learning principles when developing intervention plans and strategies.

11. In the task-oriented model, tasks can be accomplished in more than one way; individuals are encouraged to actively problem-solve and to learn alternative movement patterns that can be used in a variety of environments. The clinician's role is to provide feedback while manipulating environmental and musculoskeletal demands to help promote the emergence of smooth and efficient functional behavior.

12. Gentile suggests that goal-directed functional behavior can be analyzed at three levels: action, movements, and the neuromotor process. Motor learning at the action level is reflected not only in the motor production and movement patterns of the performer but also in the ability of the performer to execute specific tasks in distinct and varied environments. The second level of analysis focuses on analyzing the movements used to perform the functional task, whereby motor learning may be evident by the performance of new patterns of movement or by changes in the kinematics of a movement. Finally, the functional task is analyzed from the perspective of the underlying processes that contribute to the movement being performed. Remembering that functional movement emerges through the interaction of many subsystems, the contributions from each need to be recognized and described.

Table 6–6 in the workbook offers a useful guide to task analysis. See main text for details.

13. Movement strategy involves helping the patient develop multijoint coordinated movements that are effective in meeting the demands of the specific task. Sensory strategy involves helping the patient learn to effectively use sensory information to meet task demands. Compensatory strategies are alternative movement strategies that replace typical movement patterns when age-related changes or impairment prevent the use of the typical patterns of coordination. Age-related changes in movement strategies in healthy adults may contribute to slowed movement and changes in the pattern of the movement, all due to some of the musculoskeletal changes that accompany normal aging. Cognitive and perceptual strategies include how an individual appears to organize the motor, sensory, and perceptual information necessary to performing a task in different environments.

14. Compensation is a behavioral substitution where alternative behavioral strategies are adopted to accomplish a task. Recovery is the achievement of function through *original* processes, whereas compensation is achieving function through *alternative* processes. Appropriate compensations use movement patterns that resemble normal or typical movements and incorporate the involved and uninvolved body segments into the movement pattern. Undesirable compensations promote asymmetries, poor alignment in the trunk and limbs, and decreased weight acceptance and lead to inefficient or unsafe movement production.

15. Impairments present anywhere from one to combinations of limitation in any one of the systems contributing to movement production as well as multisystem impairments of posture, balance, and gait. Examples of impairments commonly associated with a neurological disorder can be muscle weakness, abnormalities of muscle tone, coordination problems, and involuntary movements.

16. Some clinical applications of the task-oriented model are as follows. Collaborate with the individual in identifying problematic tasks of interest and importance, analyze the preferred movements for task performance and the observed outcomes, record the observed changes in the preferred movements for task perform-

ance and those outcomes, and vary the environmental context and the practice conditions to facilitate learning and flexible task performance.

17. Functional training is a method of retraining the movement system using repetitive practice of functional tasks in an attempt to establish or reestablish the individual's ability to perform activities of daily living.

18. Strategies to improve mobility are based on a careful assessment regarding the apparent reason for the demonstrated lack of initial mobility. Activities should be implemented that will help gain mobility. Effective strategies to enhance stability control include the facilitation techniques described as approximation and resistance, strengthening activities to enhance proximal stability, isometrics, rhythmic stabilization, and weight-bearing activities. Strategies to improve controlled mobility include emphasis on movements with directional changes that encourage antagonist muscle actions, such as weight shifting and performing transitional movements. Skill strategies include active, goal-directed practice of specific task-oriented activities and the promotion of successful motor learning, problem solving, retaining, and transferring movements across environmental contexts within a variety of tasks.

19. Functional goals are based on the needs and desires of the individual and on the functional impairments that have been identified by the therapist during evaluation. Functional limitation (activity limitation) is a restriction of the ability to perform, at the level of the whole person, a physical action, activity, or task, in an efficient, typically expected, or competent manner. The clinical process used during intervention according to a person-centered functional goal approach involves three steps: determine the individual's desired outcome of therapy; develop an understanding of the individual's self-care, work, and leisure activities and the environments within which these activities occur; and establish and work toward mutual goals together with the patient/client.

20. Therapeutic intervention needs to include any combination of sensorimotor techniques, task-oriented analysis, functional training, and motor control/motor learning strategies to offer the individual the most appropriate and efficient route to functional independence or optimal quality of life. An integrated approach preserves the individualism of the patient/client and requires the clinician to be a current, problem-solving practitioner.

Chapter Seven

1. Muscle weakness is an inability to generate normal levels of muscular force and is a major impairment of motor function in patients/clients with nervous system damage. Muscle tone abnormalities found in patients who have upper motor neuron lesions are broad, ranging from flaccidity, or complete loss of muscle tone, to hypertonicity, or spasticity. Coordinated muscle movement involves multiple joints and muscles that are activated at the appropriate time and with the correct amount of force so that smooth, efficient, and accurate movement occurs. Coordination deficits occur when muscles fail to fire in sequence or when the central nervous system is unable to direct movement activities properly. Involuntary movements are a common sign of neurological damage and include dystonia (sustained muscle contractions), tremors (rhythmical, oscillatory movements of a body part), and athetoid and choreiform movements. Athetoid movement is slow, involuntary writhing or twisting, usually involving the upper extremities more than the lower extremities. Choreiform movement is involuntary, jerky, rapid, and irregular.

2. Positive features of brain damage are defined as abnormal behaviors due directly to the lesion, including the presence of abnormal movement patterns such as a pathological reflex response or hyperactive stretch reflex. Negative features are due to a loss or deficit of motor behavior. Examples of negative features are weakness and slowness of movement.

3. Central nervous system lesions can result in a wide variety of primary impairments affecting motor, sensory, perceptual, and cognitive systems. An example of a primary motor impairment is weakness. Secondary impairments also contribute to movement problems demonstrated by patients. Secondary impairments do not result from the central nervous system pathology directly; rather, they develop as a result of the consequences of the pathology or primary impairment. An example of a secondary impairment is loss of range of motion. Both primary and secondary impairments have an effect on functional performance.

4. Muscular weakness is an inability to generate normal levels of muscular force and is a major impairment of motor function in patients/clients with central nervous system damage. Depending on the extent of the lesion, weakness in the patient with a nervous system or upper motor neuron lesion can vary in severity from total loss to mild or partial loss of muscle activity. Weakness is often masked by the parallel symptom of spasticity. Some of the clinical consequences of weakness are impaired voluntary movement, instability, limited postural control and, ultimately, functional or activity limitation.

5. Muscle tone is a state of readiness of skeletal muscle so that the muscular system is in a state of arousal prepared for the task demands to be placed on it. Muscle tone is determined by the level of excitability of the entire pool of motor neurons controlling a muscle, the intrinsic stiffness of the muscle itself, and the level of sensitivity of many reflexes.

6. Hypotonia is a reduction in muscle stiffness, often seen in spinocerebellar lesions and in developmental disorders, such as a type of cerebral palsy or Down syndrome. Flaccidity, the most severe manifestation of hypotonia, is characterized as the complete loss of muscle tone. Patients/clients with hypotonia present with weakness, a decreased ability to sustain muscle activation, a decreased ability to coactivate muscle groups, abnormal joint mobility patterns, and a delayed or ineffective exhibition of normal postural responses.

7. Common clinical problems and functional impairments associated with hypotonia include weakness with decreased strength and decreased antigravity control, decreased ability to sustain muscle group activation evidenced by an inability to maintain postural alignment and control in static positions, fatigability, decreased ability to coactivate muscle groups evidenced by an inability to maintain postural alignment and control in static positions, susceptibility to injury, decreased postural control when displaced or while moving, poor balance, and frequent falls. Goals include increased voluntary strength: isometrically, eccentrically and concentrically, increased antigravity control in functional positions, increased muscle activation, incorporation of endurance training into functional retraining, increased co-contraction and proximal stability, appropriate functional positioning and orthotic management, and improved balance.

8. Spasticity is a symptom of a motor disorder characterized by a velocity-dependent increase in the stretch reflex with exaggerated tendon jerks, resulting from hyperexcitability. Stiffness is reflective of changes in the viscoelastic properties of the muscle tissue, often associated with contracture and additional clinical signs. Spasticity is used to describe a wide range of abnormal motor behaviors including hyperactive stretch reflexes, abnormal posturing of the limbs, excessive coactivation of the antagonist muscles, associated movements, and stereotypical movements synergies. Normal, voluntary movement control is impaired in the patient/client with spasticity.

9. There are several intervention options available for the patient/client with spasticity. Because spasticity is a symptom of impaired voluntary motor control, activities to improve voluntary movement control and strength are indicated. Decreasing spasticity is a goal of intervention when the spasticity limits that person's function. Prolonged stretch can be used to induce relaxation in a spastic muscle. Sensorimotor approaches using sensory stimulation techniques can be used to either facilitate or inhibit muscle tone, depending on the use of the stimulus and how it is applied. Changes in body position can significantly alter muscle tone or spasticity in individuals with an upper motor neuron lesion. Neurosurgical interventions include selective posterior rhizotomy and the use of an intrathecal baclofen pump. Pharmaceutical interventions, including Botox, may be indicated. Electrical stimulation to increase voluntary motor control and active muscle strength has been demonstrated to be of value.

10. The common clinical problems and functional impairments associated with hypertonicity include weakness with limited strength in movements against gravity; poor voluntary movement control; evidence of increased muscle tone predominantly in the extremities with subsequent stereotypical movements and inability to move fast and efficiently; a decreased ability to activate isolated muscle groups in the extremities (such as hip extensors, triceps) required for functional control as evidenced by inability to sustain effective weight bearing; difficulty terminating certain muscle groups (hip flexors, adductors, internal rotators) as required for

functional control, evidenced by decreased control of movement and difficulty with deceleration at end ranges; a decreased ability to stabilize a loaded joint eccentrically and a decreased ability to combine flexion and extension smoothly during posture and movement; inaccurate muscle recruitment; decreased strength in the trunk; decreased rotation and dissociation during movement; and secondary loss in range of motion with subsequent limited excursion to complete functional movement. Goals of intervention include increasing strength and voluntary, isolated movement control; activation of functional muscle patterns; increased ability to accept loading onto upper or lower extremities as required for function through isometric work and functional use of developmental positions; work on eccentric control during functional movement; increased ability to balance flexors and extensors; effective use of combinations of movements and transitions involving trunk rotation; increased accuracy of responses to postural changes and balance activities; and preventive management to decrease functional limitations caused by secondary impairments.

11. Rigidity is characterized by a heightened resistance to passive movement but independent of the velocity of that stretch or movement. Rigidity is often associated with basal ganglia pathology, such as Parkinson's disease. Lead pipe rigidity is constant resistance to movement. Cogwheel rigidity is characterized by alternate episodes of resistance and relaxation, recognizable clinically by a ratchet-like response to passive movement characterized by an alternate letting go and increased resistance to movement. Decorticate rigidity refers to the state of sustained contraction of the trunk and lower limbs in extension and of the upper limbs in flexion, indicative of a corticospinal tract lesion at the level of the diencephalon, above the superior colliculus. Decerebrate rigidity refers to a state of sustained contraction of the trunk and all four limbs into extension, indicative of a brain stem lesion.

12. Intervention to manage rigidity should be directed at enhancing functional movements and at cognitive retraining, not at focusing on the rigidity as the main impairment responsible for difficulties with functional performance. Many of the specific therapeutic interventions are similar to those listed for intervention with spasticity. Pharmacological management has also been shown to be successful.

13. Lack of coordination can impair the quality of movement or can be so severe that it limits movement altogether. Incoordination occurs when the firing rates of muscles are disrupted, resulting in loss of smooth movement, or when the central nervous system loses its ability to direct movement activity that requires accuracy. Problems with sequencing are often characterized by inappropriate coactivation, which means that the agonist and antagonist both fire, and smooth movement is impaired. Abnormal synergies are stereotypical patterns of movement that do not change or adapt to environmental or task demands. There can be many facets to timing errors, including problems initiating the movement, slowed movement execution, and problems terminating a movement.

14. Coordination problems can be clinically managed by using external cues to help guide the individual with uncoordinated movement effectively through the motor performance. Repetition and practice of a functional and task-specific movement can also help manage coordination problems. Functional strength training, work within range of motion in small increments, work on co-contraction and postural stability, and work to increase the ability to stabilize and transition with control have been found to be effective. Involuntary movements seem to decrease by directing controlled movements and increasing response accuracy to postural changes.

15. Dystonia is a syndrome dominated by sustained muscle contraction, frequently causing abnormal postures, twisting or writhing movements, and repetitive abnormal posture. Movements range from slow to quick patterns and even co-contraction of the agonist and antagonist. Tremor is a rhythmical, involuntary, oscillatory movement of a body part. Associated movements are characterized by involuntary movement of one body part during the voluntary movement of another body part. Athetoid movement is slow, involuntary writhing or twisting, usually involving the upper extremities more than the lower extremities. Choreiform movements are involuntary, jerky, rapid, and irregular. Their main clinical effects on movement control include poor voluntary motor control, lack of postural stability, inability to hold body segments at various points within the range of motion, difficulty changing positions and combining functional movements, ineffective weight bearing, instability and unsafe

movement, poor movement transitions, difficulty with midline control and symmetrical muscle action, decreased ability to realign posture when displaced or while moving, and difficulty with functional, purposeful movements.

16. The main therapeutic interventions for clinical management of involuntary movement include strength training, sensorimotor techniques, functional task training, movement reeducation, and energy conservation education. Rehabilitation strategies for treating involuntary movement focus primarily on compensating for the movement rather than on changing the movement itself.

17. The common clinical problems and functional limitations associated with dystonia are described in Answer 15. Therapy goals include functional strength training, work within range of motion in small increments, work on co-contraction and postural stability, work on trunk control and proximal stability, increased ability to sustain postures, improved co-contraction and stability, increased ability to stabilize and transition with control, increased controlled symmetry and midline postural control, improved balance, and more effective, safe, functional movement. Midline stability of the head and trunk are vital so that the individual can optimize functional, social, visual, and self-help skills. Selected techniques from many intervention approaches can be useful in facilitating maximal functional performance.

18. Problem-solving clinicians need to first identify what factor or factors seem to interfere most with motor performance. The major impairments of weakness, uncoordinated movement, and the adaptive changes of muscle stiffness and abnormal posturing are typically among the factors that interfere most with functional motor behavior. The focus is on minimizing the interfering effects of neurological damage while maximizing voluntary control. Neurological rehabilitation should begin early and be active. Functional training requires a very individualized assessment of the patient/client and an inventory of meaningful and troublesome tasks *for that person*. Encouraging the patient to be active seems to be a critical factor. Engaging the individual in meaningful, occupational-embedded tasks is crucial for success.

19. Due to the in-depth nature of this answer, the reader is referred to the text. The case studies in Chapter 7 and Tables 7–2 through 7–4 in the main text can be used as reference.

Chapter Eight

1. Postural control is the ability to maintain a steady position in a weight-bearing, antigravity posture.

2. Balance is the ability to maintain a steady position in a weight-bearing, antigravity posture while adjusting to voluntary limb movements and external/environmental disturbances.

3. Postural adjustments are subtle changes in the postural control system to reduce or eliminate a displacement of the center of gravity.

4. Postural preparations are changes made prior to the execution of a planned movement, also called anticipatory adjustments. They are used, for example, when one stiffens one's joints when ice skating for the first time.

5. Postural accompaniments are adjustments occurring at the same time as the intended movement. They are used when the conditions of the task are well known.

6. The theoretical models used to explain the neural control of posture and balance include the hierarchical model (reflex integration over time and increasing central nervous system control of movement) and systems model (interaction of several systems, characteristics of the task itself, and the environment all influence posture).

7. The righting reactions include the labyrinthine, optical, and body righting reactions. All are attempts to realign the head or body parts to each other or to the environment. They contribute to forward movement and anti-gravity positions.

8. Equilibrium reactions are body movements over the base of support or to increase the base of support; also known as the tilting reactions. They help in the development of system interaction necessary for the child to gain independence in each developmental position.

9. Orienting reactions are movements of the head

or body to bring an object into clearer vision or into reach. They lead to the development of thalamocortical connections (sensory impulses reaching the cortex for conscious attention).

10. Head control is the ability to maintain upright position of the head despite body position changes. The development and practice of head control allow for mastery of isolation of movement of body parts rather than movement in generalized patterns.

11. Postural sway influences trunk control development because movement that occurs as the musculoskeletal system adjusts to environment changes to keep the trunk upright contributes to effective postural control. Trunk control develops as sway is incorporated into the movement plan, allowing alignment.

12. An example of a musculoskeletal limitation that contributes to postural instability is loss of spinal flexibility as it contributes to immobility in patients/clients with Parkinson's disease.

13. The three neuromuscular factors that contribute to the organization of muscle forces for postural control are: postural alignment—influences the motor plan to keep the body centered about the vertical midline; muscle tone—the readiness of muscles to contract; postural tone—activation of specific antigravity muscles that stabilize weight-bearing joints and the trunk.

14. The three primary systems whose input directly affects postural control and balance are the visual, vestibular, and somatosensory systems.

15. Due to the large amount of information received quickly, vision predominates the sensory input. The consequence is that visual information is often accepted as accurate even in the presence of profound impairment.

16. The three visual projection areas include lateral geniculate nucleus of the thalamus—projections to the primary visual cortex for object identification; superior colliculus—detects movement within the visual fields and provides spatial (location) information; accessory optic tract—a feedback loop to control eye movement keeping the gaze steady.

17. Focal vision provides for recognition and identification of objects within the visual field.

Ambient vision provides for location within the field of view: "where is it?" information.

18. The major anatomical structures of the vestibular system include semicircular canals—acceleration or deceleration of rotary movements like turning the head; labyrinths—acceleration and movement deceleration of linear movements (car pulling out from a stop sign) and the effects of gravity.

19. Vestibular structures collect input and compare the information to the movement plan to provide for smooth voluntary movements. They have a direct influence on muscle tone for postural control.

20. In central vestibular disorders, projection fibers are affected, whereas in peripheral vestibular disorders, inner ear structures are affected.

21. The vestibular (ocular) reflex provides for maintenance of a steady image on the retina through regulation of eye position in the orbit influenced by information from the accessory optic tract and vestibular fibers.

22. The major anatomical structures of the peripheral system related to postural control and balance are the tactile receptors and the proprioceptors in muscle, tendons, and joints. They monitor the body position to provide feed forward preparations and trigger postural corrections

23. Perception adds meaning to the sensory impulses received by the brain from the various somatosensory receptors. An example is knowing that you have found a quarter when you feel the bumps and ridges on the edge of a round, metal object in your coin purse.

24. Body image reflects what one believes about oneself: self-image, internal representation of who one is. Body schema refers to knowledge of the position of one's body parts in relationship to each other and to the environment.

25. Laterality is an awareness of two sides of the body, right and left. Directionality provides for a sense of the direction an object is in relative to oneself in the environment.

26. The following cognitive mechanisms influence postural control and balance and treatment of imbalance. Arousal means being alert to

the environment to prepare for changes, attention directs cognitive processes to significant features in the area, memory allows a comparison to previous experience for planning or to encode novel experiences, judgment provides a mechanism for discernment of appropriateness of action choices, and decision making results in a selection of action from an array of possibilities.

27. The strategies used by the sensory system for postural stability and balance include attempts to reduce the amount of conflicting input and coordinate the sensory information with motor information/planning. The goal is to maintain posture in the absence of challenges.

28. Vertigo is a sense of movement when there is no actual position change.

29. The ankle strategy of postural recovery is postural control initiated from the ankles/feet; used to correct anterior-posterior sway or when a challenge is small, slow, or near the vertical midline.

30. The hip strategy of postural recovery is movement at the pelvis and trunk to correct posture; this results in a shift of the center of gravity due to large body movements and is the choice when the challenge is large, fast, or in the presence of a small base of support.

31. The stepping strategy of postural recovery is limb movement to increase the base of support and is used when the challenge is very large or very fast; the strategy allows the center of mass to realign with the base of support by increasing the size of the center of mass.

32. Controlled movement occurs within the current base of support, whereas skilled movements reach to the extremes of the support base.

33. Reactive control is movement made in response to ongoing feedback; preparations for movement relative to current task and environmental conditions are anticipatory.

34. The major challenges to developing postural control in early development include gaining proximal muscle control to stabilize the body so segments are free to move/function, learning to isolate movement, and conquering the force of gravity.

35. The major challenges to developing postural control in childhood include widening the range of stability movements, relearning strategies as the body grows and develops, and learning skilled movements to use as a stable frame for future movement.

36. The major challenges to developing postural control in adolescence include application of movement strategies to a particular sport or activity of daily living. Movement becomes more a function of self-expression and is refined for personal preferences during this age stage.

37. The major challenges to developing postural control in adulthood are task-in-context interaction (learning performance is dependent on system interaction) and smooth use of righting and equilibrium responses.

38. The musculoskeletal changes that occur with age that greatly affect postural control and balance are decreases in muscle strength, range of motion, and spinal flexibility; vertical alignment undergoes a posterior shift.

39. The neuromuscular change that occurs with age that affects postural control and balance is a decrease in the control and coordination of muscle.

40. Tactile stimulus sensitivity decreases; vibratory sensation is lost, peripheral vision is lost, and the integrity of each system decreases.

41. The cognitive changes that result from aging, which affect postural control and balance, are that more attention is required in a novel environment, which decreases attention to postural control mechanisms.

42. Some commonly used functional balance assessments are the Timed Get Up and Go test, which gives a practical examination of functional balance, and Functional Reach, which relates to risk of falls, especially in elderly.

43. Commonly used assessments of balance systems are Romberg's test, which differentiates cerebellar influence on posture; the postural stress test, which is a reliable push test demonstrating the recoverable amount of challenge, and the Clinical Test for Sensory Integration in Balance, which tests for separate sensory system influence on the observed balance problem. See the text for details.

44. Impairment intervention focuses on the part or system causing the problem; strategy intervention leads to the development of new or different strategies to employ when a challenge is encountered; functional treatment/intervention focuses on the demands of everyday activities where difficulty is most likely to be encountered.

45. Some of the techniques used to address remediation of balance dysfunction at the impairment level include sensory reeducation, vestibular rehabilitation, and musculoskeletal strengthening.

46. Some of the techniques used to address remediation of balance dysfunction at the strategy level include task analysis and adaptation to encourage use of an alternate system to assess postural stability.

47. Functional level of task performance refers to the real-life experience of a balance problem and considers ways to make corrections focusing on the demands of the task rather than on the body systems. Postural adjustments appear to be task-specific; for transfer-of-training, the real-life experience of imbalance is required.

Chapter Nine

1. In the early stages of development, the upper extremity is involved in closed chain activities to help provide stability through the shoulder such as weight bearing in quadruped and in prone. As the infant grows and develops, the upper extremity is used to help gain sensory information by exploring objects as well as the infant's own body. Haptic perception is developed, which enhances the infant's ability to manipulate and grasp. By the end of the first year of life, the infant has a voluntary reach and grasp and is able to use refined pincer grasp and a controlled release of objects. During the early childhood years, the functional tasks of the upper extremity during reach and grasp are refined to allow the child to master skills such as self-feeding, tool use, and dressing. In-hand manipulative skills needed for writing and other fine motor activities are a focus of the elementary school–aged child. Functional tasks of the upper extremity including anticipatory grasp and controlled release, which are needed for sporting activities, playing a musical instrument, and prevocational skills in the adolescent increase and are soon similar to those of an adult. In adulthood, functional tasks of the upper extremity such as grip strength and manipulative skills can be increased or maintained through practice and use. As the adult ages, however, normal changes in body systems such as decreased flexibility and strength begin to hamper upper extremity skills such as reach and grasp.

2. Somatosensory input is initially used by the upper extremity as a survival system as seen in primitive reflexes. As the individual matures, proprioception and tactile information are vital for development of haptic perception, controlled movements of the hand, and in-hand manipulation. Somatosensory input allows one to determine how to vary grip strengths and manipulate different objects for functional use and also provides important input needed for anticipatory control. Proprioceptive input is also important during reach in providing information needed to position the upper extremity in space and allow the reach pattern to be smooth and precise.

3. After the first few months of life, vision initiates overall movement in the infant. Vision is used during the phase of regard in which the individual visually regards an object and is able to fix and follow the object. Successful reach depends, in part, on visual feedback, which allows the individual to fine-tune the upper extremities' approach to the object. Vision is also important input used during anticipatory control. This ability to form motor memories is based on visual and somatosensory input and allows an individual to adapt reach and grasp patterns.

4. Power grasp occurs when the whole hand is used to grasp something, with the thumb held close to the other digits. Stability throughout the proximal musculature, such as the shoulder girdle and the wrist and forearm, is needed to successfully grasp and lift large objects. Precision grasp is one in which the thumb is held in opposition. Rotation of the thumb provided through the wide range of movement and stability of the carpometacarpal joint are needed for a successful precision grasp. Intact in-hand manipulation skills and sensory systems are also needed.

5. Examples of power grasp include picking up a grocery bag with handles, opening a large jar, and turning a key in a lock. Examples of precision grasp include holding a needle for

sewing, holding a pencil, and grasping a tennis ball.

6. A lateral pinch is used when the lateral aspects of the fingers hold the object (such as how a hairdresser holds the hair between his or her fingers in order to cut it); a two-point pinch requires the use of two finger pads, usually the thumb and index finger (such as holding a tack or push pin); and a three-point pinch requires the use typically of the thumb, index, and middle finger.

7. The infant begins reaching behaviors as visually guided movements in which objects are swiped at and randomly contacted. By 4 to 5 months, the infant is able to use vision, sensory input, and upper body stability to reach a target. As the infant is able to sit independently and attain a variety of upright positions, his or her ability to reach in different planes increases. By 9 months, the infant is able to reach for an object in a smooth and coordinated manner and continues to refine and practice this skill throughout the first year of life. Initially, the infant is able to grasp, using proprioceptive and tactile input to initiate a reflexive grasp. By 3 to 5 months, voluntary grasping emerges, and between 4 and 5 months, the infant is able to orient his or her hand to an object. Early exploration of objects begins at this age as does midline orientation of objects. Haptic perception and the foundation for in-hand manipulation skills begin during the early stages of development. During grasping the thumb initially is in an adducted position. By 7 to 9 months, more opposition of the thumb emerges, with refined opposition allowing tip-to-tip pinch of the index finger and thumb to occur by 12 months.

8. Anticipatory control allows the use of past experiences and sensory perceptions to form sensory motor memories that allow adaptation of reach and grasp. An example is reaching for a glass. The person's hand begins to form in the shape of the glass prior to grasping it.

9. Haptic perception is the ability to use tactile and proprioceptive information to discriminate different attributes of an object. This perception allows the development and refinement of grasp patterns and manipulative skills. Therefore the haptic qualities of an object tend to produce different grasping patterns.

10. The components needed to develop in-hand manipulation skills include coordination of the

sensory systems used in grasp, haptic perception, forearm supination, wrist stability, refined thumb and index movement, dissociation of the two sides of the hand, and volition. The foundation for these skills begins during the first year of life and begins to emerge during the preschool years.

11. Translation is the ability to move an object to and from the palm from and to the fingertips, such as moving a coin from the palm to the fingertips to place it in a vending machine. Shift is when an object is moved or adjusted on the fingertips, such as adjusting the handle of a spoon along the fingertips. Rotation can be simple or complex and involves rolling or turning an object along the fingertips with the thumb in opposition, such as turning the dial on a combination lock or turning a marker over to remove the cap.

12. There are many changes that affect the normal adult during the aging process that hinder the functional skills of the upper extremity. Some of these changes include decreased visual acuity and visual processing and presence of cataracts; decreased muscle mass and synaptic firing; decreased bone mass and changes in articular cartilage; and somatosensory changes including decreased proprioception and tactile discrimination.

13. During regard, the individual with weakness may be unable to position his or her head appropriately to locate and track the object he or she is reaching for. Oculomotor movements may also be affected in this individual. Weakness hinders reach by decreasing shoulder stability and range of movement. Fatigue and the inability to hold the arm in certain positions during the reaching phase can also lead to incorrect placement of the hand for grasp. Once an object is in the hand, decreased grasp strength and endurance during pinch activities and in-hand manipulation skills can make everyday functional activities difficult for the individual with weakness. Controlled release of objects can also be affected in these individuals in whom precision and timing for release of objects are decreased.

14. The client with abnormal muscle tone can exhibit decreased ability to regard an object due to inability to position the head correctly. Visual problems often seen in these clients can also hinder the ability to visually regard objects. During reach, the client with low muscle tone may have many of the limitations described

earlier due to lack of glenohumeral stability. Conversely, increased muscle tone can cause limited active range of motion of the shoulder and hampered timing and control during reaching. During grasp and manipulation, abnormal muscle tone affects the balance between the muscles of the hand, making in-hand manipulation skills difficult. The somatosensory system, also important in grasping and manipulation, can be impaired in an individual with abnormal muscle tone, leading to decreases in these functional tasks.

15. Incoordination often hinders smooth visual pursuits and eye-head coordination needed for regarding objects. During the reaching phase, individuals with incoordination have poor accuracy and timing and often use many movement segments rather than one smooth movement. Incoordination can cause decreased ability to adjust grip forces and lack of fluid in-hand movements during grasp, manipulation, and release. For example, individuals who suffer from basal ganglia lesions also have decreased ability initiating grasp and release skills.

16. Individuals with cerebral palsy often have visual and perceptual deficits, which can lead to decreased ability to visually regard, track, or maintain visual fixation on an object. Poor postural control can also limit head-neck control and lead to an inadequate visual foundation for perceptual learning. Limited postural control and abnormal muscle tone in the upper extremity and supportive musculature can cause a deficit in postural stability and limit the availability of varied distal strategies for reach and grasp. During the grasp and manipulation phase of object exploration, individuals with cerebral palsy often have limited processing of sensory information needed for these skills, specifically tactile and proprioceptive input. Some grasp and manipulation problems observed in children with cerebral palsy include exaggerated opening and closing of the hand, decreased ability to grade grip forces, poor differentiation between ulnar and radial sides of the hand, and lack of precision and inaccuracy with small hand movements. During the release phase, wrist flexion and finger extension is often seen as this pattern offers a mechanical advantage. Limited control in finger and wrist extensors as well as decreased proprioceptive feedback often causes this inefficient pattern.

17. Some of the most common therapeutic interven-

tions available for the clinical management of upper extremity dysfunction as seen in the individual with cerebral palsy include weight bearing on the upper extremity in different developmental positions such as prone on elbows or quadruped, reaching while participating in an activity is one strategy that the therapist can use to work on building stability through the shoulder girdle and head and neck; a graded reaching activity such as starting in a gravity-eliminated plane like side lying may be helpful for children with hypotonia. Side lying is a good position because it provides some proximal stability and encourages hand in a midline orientation within the visual field. Weight bearing, traction, and vibration may be helpful in decreasing spasticity during intervention sessions. Using different toys and objects with varied sensory attributes (texture, weight, size) can also help to provide more input and experience for the child during the grasp and manipulation phase. The size and shape of the object should be appropriate for the grasp pattern the therapist is working on with the child. Specialized equipment such as seating to provide outside stability or splints to help decrease muscle tone or provide support may be needed to facilitate the individual's upper extremity goals.

18. Many clients have visual problems following a cerebrovascular accident. These problems, along with decreased head and trunk stability and possible disorientation and agitation, can cause a decrease in the person's ability to regard an object. During the reaching phase, there are many possible problems with the shoulder girdle that are common. Decreased alignment of the glenohumeral joint, unbalanced muscle activation, and pain are just some of the factors that limit reach in these individuals. One of the common reaching patterns in individuals post–cerebrovascular accident is shoulder elevation and adduction, internal rotation and elbow, wrist and finger flexion. Impaired sensation on the involved side is also a factor affecting reach. Factors such as decreased sensation, joint changes, poor shoulder girdle alignment, weakness or paralysis, and imbalances in muscle pull can cause difficulty during grasp and manipulation. Poor ability to grasp and manipulate objects and prevalent patterns of wrist flexion and finger flexion are often seen. Varying muscle tone along with sensory losses in the hand hinder timing and graded release in clients with cerebrovascular accident. This can cause an

inability to release objects, with the individual having to pry the object out of the involved hand. Likewise, patients/clients can have an inability to sustain a grasp, causing everything to drop from their hand.

19. Visual neglect or inattention on the involved side of the individual with cerebrovascular accident is a common problem affecting the ability to regard and visually attend to objects. Therapists and assistants may use strategies such as verbally cuing the patient/client to visually scan the environment or use visual imagery. During reach, trunk alignment should be facilitated if possible during functional activities such as dressing. Alignment of the scapula and shoulder girdle is also important for the patient with hemiplegia in the upper extremity. Weight bearing in different positions can start to strengthen shoulder stabilizers as well as decrease muscle tone if abnormally high. Pain and edema are also common components observed in the patient with cerebrovascular accident and should be addressed. Edema in the early stages can be decreased through elevation, gentle active motion, and retrograde massage. Pain also hinders functional movement and should be addressed early in the attempt to avoid chronic pain syndromes. A detailed list of intervention strategies is listed in the text. Some of the common goals for increasing grasp and manipulation include providing joint alignment; increasing range of motion; decreasing edema, pain, and spasticity; and improving voluntary movement and strength. Grasping often begins with the establishment of a voluntary power grasp. This is followed by working on more precise pinch patterns. The clinician must be mindful of the attributes of the objects being grasped as these influence grasp patterns. Grasp and manipulation activities that have meaning to the individual versus rote exercise provide a better outcome. For example, grasping a spoon for eating versus placing pegs in a pegboard has more intrinsic value to an individual and should be incorporated into intervention. For individuals who have difficulty initiating release due to spasticity, techniques such as vibration, tapping, or slow sustained stretch may be used to help begin the release process. Adaptive equipment such as reachers and one-handed devices may be helpful in increasing the independence of the individual with cerebrovascular accident.

20. The individual with Parkinson's disease can have a variety of visual deficits, which can limit the ability to visually regard objects. These deficits include blurry vision, impaired saccadic eye movements, and decreased acuity. Because the visual system is often used to override the motor system in the individual with Parkinson's disease, visual disturbances should be addressed. Movements during reach are hindered, especially when multiple joints are used. The hallmarks of Parkinson's disease include rigidity, bradykinesia, and akinesia. These movement disturbances can cause the patient/client to have limited ability to reach for objects due to a paucity of movement. Grasp and manipulation often involve multiple joints and steps and therefore are very difficult for the patient. Lack of graded grip force, increased time in generating a grasping motion, and limited manipulative skills are common. During the release phase, the patient may have difficulty initiating release, especially if increased speed is needed.

21. External cues including verbal, visual, tactile, and proprioceptive can help assist the patient/client with Parkinson's disease in performing motor sequences. Examples of visual cues include dark, lined paper or raised line paper to help alleviate handwriting difficulties. Rocking to help a client get out of bed is an example of a proprioceptive cue that may assist with initiating a motor sequence. Verbal cues are commonly used, such as "left arm up" and must be very simple and concise. Breaking tasks into smaller components is another strategy that can assist the individual with Parkinson's disease who has difficulty initiating multistep tasks. Finally, adaptive equipment may also be helpful.

Chapter Ten

1. The main functional tasks of the lower extremities include the ability to support body weight on both legs, to transfer weight from one leg to the other, to bear weight on one leg and then move the other leg, and to constantly adapt to movements of the trunk and upper extremities. Lower extremity capabilities allow for all of the functions of moving the body through space, including all of the locomotor skills of rolling, crawling and creeping, walking, running, skipping, and hopping. Functionally, the main task of the lower extremities is more often concerned with weight bearing, stability, and mobility, including all of the gross motor activities that accomplish the task of locomotion through

space: rolling, crawling and creeping, and walking. However, lower extremity function in non–weight-bearing is also important for full independent function.

2. Non–weight-bearing functions of the lower extremities are movements of the extremity in space, often referred to as open chain activities. Non–weight-bearing movements of the lower extremity have important functional uses. The swing phase of gait or flexion of the leg to go up a step or engage in a dressing activity are examples. Weight-bearing occurs when the extremities are stabilized against a surface in a position where they support body weight and form part of the body's base of support, such as during stance or gait.

3. Non–weight-bearing movements are used functionally to position the extremity for task performance, to execute the movement patterns required by the task, and to return the extremity from this functional position to rest against the body. Non–weight-bearing movements of the lower extremities are vitally important in many positions, including the functional positions of sitting and standing. In sitting, non–weight-bearing lower extremity movements are those movements used in sitting to change body position or to engage in activities of daily living. In standing, to move the non–weight-bearing leg forward, alignment and control of the trunk, trunk and pelvic stability, and sequenced muscle activation patterns all allow the leg to move forward. Any limitation in the functional movements required to perform these tasks, secondary to immobility, weakness, or interference from abnormal muscle tone, may result in a functional limitation requiring intervention.

4. During weight-bearing activities, the lower extremity muscles are active to maintain a stable contact with the supporting surface, to maintain good alignment over distal segments, and to lift and support the weight of the body against the force of gravity. The most common lower extremity weight-bearing tasks are movement activation required for stance control and ambulation. Any limitation in the functional movements required to perform these tasks, secondary to immobility, weakness, or interference from abnormal muscle tone, may result in a functional limitation requiring intervention.

5. Functional upright stance control is important for balance and safety in standing, during upper extremity tasks, and while walking. During stance, the lower extremity needs to respond to weight shifts initiated by the lower extremities and those initiated by the trunk. In both instances, the muscles of the lower extremity are activated to maintain stability and balance. Independent, safe standing is an important functional goal for most patients/clients, requiring the ability to control the lower extremities and trunk in standing. It requires lower extremity strength, alignment, muscle firing, and sequencing patterns as well as postural control for movement initiation, balance, and adaptation during functional performance. Some of the guidelines useful for directing intervention efforts to the establishment of functional upright stance control are as follows: The base of support is small, and the center of gravity is high; there is minimal postural sway; postural stability is maintained by normal postural alignment; and postural stability is maintained by minimal but important muscular activity. Postural stability in upright stance is maintained by normal postural alignment and supported by minimal but important muscular activity: in the antigravity paraspinal extensor muscles of the trunk, abdominals, gluteus maximus, hamstrings, and soleus muscles. Hip abductors are important for lateral stability. See text for further details.

6. Locomotion is the process of moving from one place to another. Locomotion is a *variable* skill in that the movement form will differ depending on the goal and the particular movement solution needed to meet that particular goal. Locomotion includes rolling, crawling, creeping, walking, galloping, skipping, hopping, and transferring from one surface to another.

7. Rolling is an important functional task and remains an important mobility skill throughout an individual's lifetime. It allows an individual to move from prone to supine and supine to prone, usually involving some amount of rotation. The most significant difference in childhood versus adult rolling is that, during infancy, the development of a mature rolling pattern closely follows the emergence and development of functional movement components. Rolling patterns develop, change, and mature as the infant exhibits increasing mastery in antigravity extensor and flexor strength, increasing dissociation both of the extremities from each other and the head and trunk from the extremities, and the emergence of smooth rotational patterns during movement. During adulthood, rotation and

dissociation continue to be evident, but the pattern used by the adult may differ depending on upper body strength versus lower body strength, abdominal and trunk strength, and whether the individual has any limitation in flexibility.

8. Crawling is progression in the prone position where the belly is in contact with the supporting surface, and the extremities are used in a reciprocal fashion to propel the body forward or backward. Creeping is progression in quadruped where the belly is lifted off the supporting surface, and the extremities move reciprocally to move the body forward and backward.

9. Kinematics is the term used to describe movement patterns such as direction of movement or joint angles without regard for the forces involved in producing the movement. Kinetics is the term used to describe the forces involved in a movement, such as muscular force. The gait cycle includes both stance and swing phase, each composed of specific functional subphases, all subservient to functional and efficient upright bipedal walking. Stance is the phase in the gait cycle when the lower extremity is in contact with the floor and is composed of the five subphases of initial contact, loading, midstance, terminal stance, and preswing. Swing phase is the phase in the gait cycle when the lower extremity is not in contact with the floor and is composed of the three subphases of initial swing, midswing, and terminal swing. Initial contact and loading are two subphases primarily responsible for stability and shock absorption. Midstance occurs when a single limb supports the body's mass requiring postural control, stability, and balance. Terminal stance involves the generation of mechanical energy to enable forward motion of the body through space and the beginning of limb advancement. Preswing functions to generate sufficient force to clear the foot from the ground. During initial swing and midswing, the limb is flexed in order to functionally shorten the limb to clear the floor. Terminal swing is characterized by a rapid extension at the knee, effectively lengthening the limb to accomplish advancement and to form a rigid lever in preparation for landing.

10. During the stance phase, the main functions are weight acceptance, loading and stabilization of the limb, energy absorption, and propulsion of the limb into the swing phase. Throughout the swing phase, the main functions are control of the momentum, limb advancement, and preparation again for stance. All of the subtasks of gait are very important to the clinician, demonstrated by the patient's ability to demonstrate stable stance, unilateral lower extremity limb loading, unweighting and advancement of a lower extremity, effective shortening of a limb for floor clearance, effective propulsion of the limb from stance into swing, and transfer of the weight to the forward advanced limb. Functional task-oriented intervention attempts to use these subphases and their correlative tasks as a framework for therapy.

11. The functional requirements of the subphases of gait can be summarized as detailed in Table 10–3 and in the following summary table (see next page).

12. The immature gait of children is typically characterized by a wide-based gait, stepping initiated primarily at the hips while keeping the knees fairly stiff, and short steps with increased periods of double support, compared with that of adults. The understanding of the development of gait, the characteristics of immature versus mature gait, and the determinants of efficient gait offers the clinician a framework for evaluating gait dysfunction in children.

13. The attributes of mature gait are as follows: stability in stance, sufficient foot clearance in swing, appropriate prepositioning of the foot during swing for initial contact, adequate step length, and efficient use of energy. Several characteristics of mature gait include pelvic tilt and rotation, initial contact with a heel strike, knee flexion at midstance, a mature relationship between mechanisms at the hip, knee, and ankle, a mature base of support, and reciprocal arm swing. It is important for the clinician to realize that mature gait does not magically appear but rather develops over time. It is also important to realize that mature gait will emerge when the prerequisites of normal gait are present. Intervention can be guided with a functional, task-oriented approach by offering opportunity for the gait prerequisites to emerge or reemerge.

14. Some gait characteristics common to older adults include a wider base of support, decreased reciprocal arm swing, and slower cadence. Stride length decreases and time in double support increases. For effective intervention, it is important that the clinician realize what may be causing the gait disorder and what

Phase	Joint Angle Requirement	Prime Muscular Force
Initial Contact	Ankle: 90° Knee: 3°–5° flexion Hip: 30° flexion	Tibialis anterior Quadriceps and hamstrings Gluteus maximus and medius
Loading	Ankle: 15° plantarflexion Knee: up to 15° flexion Hip: 30° flexion	Tibialis anterior Quadriceps Gluteus maximus
Midstance	Ankle: from 15° plantarflexion to 15° dorsiflexion Knee: 5° flexion Hip: full extension	Gastrocnemius and soleus Gluteus maximus Gluteus medius, minimus, and tensor fascia lata
Terminal Stance	Ankle: 15° dorsiflexion to 20° plantarflexion Knee: moves into full extension Hip: 10° extension	Gastrocnemius
Preswing	Ankle: 20° plantarflexion Knee: 40° flexion Hip: 10° extension	Gastrocnemius Hip adductors Rectus femoris
Initial Swing	Ankle: to neutral dorsiflexion Knee: 40°–60° flexion Hip: from extension to 30° flexion	Tibialis anterior Quadriceps Iliopsoas
Midswing	Ankle: neutral Knee: 60° flexion Hip: 30° flexion	Tibialis anterior Iliopsoas
Terminal Swing	Ankle: neutral Knee: to full extension Hip: 30° flexion	Tibialis anterior Gluteus maximus and hamstrings

steps can be taken to improve the efficiency, effectiveness, or safety of a patient's gait.

15. When using an assistive or an orthotic device, the function of the upper extremities is different during gait. The upper extremities are no longer able to engage in a reciprocal arm swing, the demands on the trunk consequently change, the ability of the trunk to freely rotate decreases, and the arms are now actually a part of the gait cycle. The use of an assistive or orthotic device will also alter the requirements of the lower extremities.

16. Weakness results in the inability to generate sufficient force to meet the demands of lower extremity control, including all locomotor skills. Abnormally low or high muscle tone may clinically present itself with the same functional limitations as caused by weakness. Abnormally high muscle tone results in several functional deficits that impair locomotor abilities, especially gait. Incoordination in lower extremity function can result from pathologic conditions in a wide variety of neural structures, including the motor cortex, basal ganglia, and cerebellum. Incoordination will affect the timing, sequencing, and efficiency of a person's gait.

17. Weakness results in the inability to generate sufficient force to meet the demands of lower extremity control, including all locomotor skills, including but not limited to walking. The functional limitations caused by muscle weakness depend on what muscles are weak, the extent of the weakness, and the capacity for other muscles to substitute for the weak muscles in meeting the requirements of the task.

18. Abnormally high muscle tone, especially spasticity, results in several functional deficits that impair locomotor abilities, especially gait. Spasticity impairs mobility in any one or any combination of five different ways:
    - Causing an overreaction to stretch and velocity-dependent movements
    - Impaired selective control
    - Inappropriate activation, sequencing, and muscle-phasing patterns
    - Abnormal movement patterns become increasingly apparent
    - Proprioception is altered

Spasticity results in the inappropriate activation of muscles during movements, including the gait cycle. This is especially problematic when muscles are undergoing lengthening during the movement task. Spasticity obstructs the yielding quality of an eccentric muscle contraction. A quick stretch can produce clonus. Spasticity in a given muscle group will contribute to a persistent firing pattern instead of an efficient burst of force, followed by a smooth decrease in activation. Spasticity also alters the mechanical properties of a muscle, producing increased stiffness, which then affects the freedom of body segments to move rapidly. This alters the smooth relationship of limb segments to each other and limits the transfer of momentum during movement (including rolling, transfers, and gait), ultimately altering the components of the task.

19. Ataxia is a common manifestation of uncoordinated control of the lower extremities, characterized by wide-based movements of the extremities. Movement decomposition is characterized by a breakdown of movements between multiple joints, resulting in movement of individual segments rather than movement as a fluid, coordinated unit. Dysmetria is characterized by overshooting, under-reaching, or reaching inaccurately toward the target, sometimes referred to as past pointing. Coactivation is inability to recruit a muscle effectively, increased activation of that muscle, or inability to modulate that muscle's activity throughout the movement.

20. Neurological pathology can lead to a wide range of secondary problems including muscular atrophy, immobility, deconditioning, joint contractures, degenerative joint disease or joint instability, and osteoporosis. Loss of flexibility, abnormal range of motion (hypomobility and hypermobility), malalignment, and muscle imbalances can result. Pain can accompany any one of these musculoskeletal impairments. Contributory interferences from any of these secondary impairments, as well as deficits in cognitive processing or perceptual abilities, must be assimilated into the therapist's assessment of the composite functional picture of the patient/client.

21. The gait patterns of individuals with neurological dysfunction are influenced primarily by deficits in force production, abnormalities of muscle tone, incoordination affecting the timing and sequencing of muscular activation patterns, and interference from involuntary movements. Functionally, these impairments may contribute to weakness, disordered motor control, immature or ineffective movement patterns, and inefficiency. Pathological gait is frequently

characterized by the following functional deficits:
- Loss of stability in stance
- Insufficient foot clearance during swing
- Inappropriate prepositioning of the foot during swing for initial contact
- Inadequate step length
- Inefficiency and poor conservation of energy

Regardless of underlying pathological condition, age, or constellation of impairments, the individual engaged in gait training is focused on establishing or reestablishing any one of the three main functional subtasks of gait, which are: weight acceptance, single limb support, and limb advancement.

22. Some of the main pathokinematic differences of gait in children with cerebral palsy are as follows: mechanical changes in spastic muscle fibers; abnormal sagittal plane motion of the knee; amplitude on EMG is lower, indicative of weakness; and lack of dorsiflexion frequently impairs the smooth movement of the tibia over the talus and may act as a brake on the forward movement of the trunk. Intervention for gait difficulties in children with cerebral palsy requires facilitation of smooth, functional movement components and integration of functional movement patterns into both preambulatory and gait activities. See text for details.

23. The main pathokinematic characteristics observed in individuals who have hemiplegia are as follows: a tendency for the flexor muscles to be active primarily during swing and the extensor muscles to be active primarily during stance in patients who demonstrate pattern-only motor control, a tendency for premature and continued activity of the stance muscles, and a tendency for co-contraction and coactivation patterns. The key to intervention for gait difficulties with patients who have experienced a stroke is to view the whole body as it cooperates during the gait cycle and to view gait as one functional movement pattern. See text for details.

24. The main pathokinematic characteristics of gait for an individual with Parkinson's disease include difficulty with initiation and momentum; hip, knee, and ankle motions are reduced with a generalized lack of extension at the hip and knee; dorsiflexion at the ankle and trunk and pelvic motions are diminished; stride length is decreased; and the patient is often observed to walk with small, shuffling steps. During inter-

vention, it is important to vary the practice of movement skills within and across varying environment contexts. Individuals will perform better if the environment is familiar and if cognitive attention to the actual movement task is shifted from the movement to the actual, familiar task. See text for details.

25. Individuals with ataxia often present with incoordination, tremor, and disturbances of posture, balance, and gait. Intervention is directed at promoting postural stability, accuracy of limb movements, and functional balance and gait. In intervention, problems with muscle firing and timing are retrained with the stance limb forward to replicate the demands of the swing cycle. The use of proximal or distal weights may assist in decreasing the ataxic movement, assisting with accuracy of swing. Remember that carryover into walking may not occur unless opportunity is given for practice within the whole, naturally occurring task of walking. Practice is offered to move smoothly from preswing into a controlled flexion and advancement of the moving limb. See text for details.

26. Spinal spasticity, resulting from a noncongenital spinal cord injury, can be quite extreme, with a characteristic distribution in the extensor muscles of the lower extremities, often with severe episodes of muscle spasm. Research suggests that this increased muscle tone may be the result of residual influence of supraspinal centers, such as the cortex, on the spinal cord and ineffective modulation of spinal pathways. The clinical result in this instance is flaccidity at the exact level of the lesion and spasticity below the level of the lesion. Spinal spasticity usually results in severe episodes of muscle spasms. A congenital spinal cord injury is associated with the most severe form of spina bifida, a condition known as myelomeningocele, in which the spinal cord and meninges of a developing fetus are contained in a sac external to the vertebral column. The clinical result is a sensory and motor impairment at the level of the lesion and below, presenting as a flaccid paralysis.

References

Allum, J., Bloem, B., Carpenter, M., Hulliger, M. & Hadders-Algra, M. (1998). Proprioceptive control of posture: a review of new concepts. Gait Posture, 8, 214–242.

American Occupational Therapy Association. (2002). Occupational therapy practice framework: domain and process. Bethesda, Md: author.

American Physical Therapy Association. (1997). Guide to physical therapist practice. Phys Ther, 77, 1163–1165

American Physical Therapy Association. (2001). Guide to physical therapist practice, ed 2. Phys Ther, 81(1).

Arend, S., & Higgins, J.R. (1976). A strategy for the classification, subjective analysis, and observation of human movement. Journal of human movement studies, 2, 36–52.

Avers, D.L. & Gardner, D.L. (2000). Patient education as a treatment modality. In Guccione, A.A. (ed.). Geriatric Physical Therapy, ed. 2. St. Louis: Mosby–Year Book.

Bear, M.F., Connors, B.W. & Paradiso, M.A. (2001). Neuroscience: Exploring the Brain, ed. 2. Baltimore: Lippincott Williams & Wilkins.

Bennett S.E., & Karnes, J.L. (1998). Neurological disabilities: Assessment and treatment. Philadelphia: Lippincott-Raven.

Breslin, D.M.M. (1996). Motor-learning theory and the neurodevelopmental treatment approach: a comparative analysis. Occup Ther Health Care, 10, 1996.

Carr, R. & Shepherd, J. (1987). A Motor Relearning Programme for Stroke. Rockville, Md: Aspen Publishers.

Carr, R. & Shepherd, J. (1998). Neurological Rehabilitation: Optimizing Motor Performance. Oxford: Butterworth Heinemann.

Cech, D. & Martin, S. (1995). Functional Movement Development Across the Life Span. Philadelphia: W.B. Saunders.

Cohen, H. (1999). Neuroscience for Rehabilitation, ed. 2. Philadelphia: Lippincott Williams & Wilkins.

Craik, R.L. (1991). Abnormalities of motor behavior. In Lister, M. (ed.). Contemporary Management of Motor Control Problems. Proceedings of the II-Step Conference, Alexandria, Va, Foundation for Physical Therapy. Fredericksburg, Va: Bookcrafters Inc.

Craik, R.L. & Oatis, C.A. (1995). Gait Analysis: Theory and Application. Philadelphia: Mosby–Year Book.

Crutchfield, C.A. & Barnes, M.R. (1993). Motor Control and Motor Learning in Rehabilitation. Atlanta: Stokesville Publishing Company.

Dunn, R., Dunn, K. & Price, G.E. (1981). Learning Style Inventory. Lawrence, Kan: Price Systems Inc.

Field-Fote, E.C. (2000). Spinal cord control of movement: implications for locomotor rehabilitation following spinal cord injury. Phys Ther, 80(5), 477–482.

Fisher, A.G. & Bundy, A.C. (1982). Equilibrium reactions in normal children and boys with sensory integration dysfunction. Occupat Ther J Res, 2, 171–183.

Flinn, N. (1995). A task-oriented approach to the treatment of a client with hemiplegia. Am J Ther, 49(6), 560–569.

Ford-Smith, C.D. & Van Sant, A. (1993). Age differences in movement patterns used to rise from a bed in subjects in the third though fifth decades of age. Phys Ther, 73(5), 300–309.

Frank, J. & Earl, M. (1990). Coordination of posture and movement. Phys Ther, 70(12), 109–117.

Gentile, A.M. (1992). The nature of skill acquisition: therapeutic implications for children with movement disorders. In Forssberg, H. & Hirschfeld, H. (eds.). Movement Disorders in Children. Med Sport Sci. Basel: Karger.

Haines, D.E. (ed.). (1997). Fundamental Neuroscience. New York: Churchill Livingstone.

Higgins, S. (1985). Movement as an emergent form: its structural limits. Hum Movement Sci, 4, 119–148.

Horak, F. (1991). Assumptions underlying motor control for neurologic rehabilitation. In Lister, M. (ed.). Contemporary Management of Motor Control Problems. Proceedings of the II-Step Conference. Alexandria, Va: Foundation for Physical Therapy. Fredericksburg, Va: Bookcrafters Inc.

Horak, F. & Nashner, M. (1986). Central programming of postural movements: adaptation to altered support-surface configurations. J Neurophysiol, 55(6), 1369–1381.

Israelevitz, T.A., Fisher, A.G. & Bundy, A.C. (1985). Equilibrium reactions in preschoolers. Occupat Ther J Res, 5(3), 154–169.

Jarus, T. (1994). Motor learning and occupational therapy: the organization of practice. Am J Ther, 48(9), 810–816.

Jette, A. M. (1994). Physical disablement concepts for physical therapy research and practice. Phys Ther, 74, 380–386.

Kamm, K., Thelen, E. & Jensen, J.L. (1990). A dynamical systems approach to motor development. Phys Ther, 70, 763–775.

Knott, M. & Voss, D.E. (1968). Proprioceptive Neuromuscular Techniques: Patterns and Techniques, ed. 2. New York: Harper & Row Publishers.

Kolb, D.A. (1999). Learning Style Inventory, ed. 3. Boston: Hay/McBer Training Resources Group, Experience Based Learning Systems, Inc.

Leonard, C.T. (1994). Major behavior and neural changes following perinatal and adult-onset brain damage: implications for therapeutic interventions. Phys Ther, 74 (8), 753–767.

Leonard, C. T. (1998). The Neuroscience of Human Movement. St. Louis: Mosby–Year Book.

Littell, E. (1990). Basic Neuroscience for the Health Professions. Thorofare, NJ: Slack, Inc.

Lundy-Ekman, L. (1998). Neuroscience: Fundamentals for Rehabilitation. Philadelphia: W.B. Saunders.

Martin, S. & Kessler, M. (2000). Neurologic Intervention for Physical Therapist Assistants. Philadelphia: W.B. Saunders.

McCormack, D.B. & Perrin, K.R. (1997). Spatial, Temporal, and Physical Analysis of Motor Control: A Comprehensive Guide to Reflexes and Reactions. San Antonio, Tex: Therapy Skill Builders.

McKeough, D.M. (1999). Neuroscience review of stroke: typical patterns. In Royeen, C.B. Neuroscience and Occupation: Links to Practice. Bethesda, Md: American Occupational Therapy Association.

Morris, M.E. (2000). Movement disorders in people with Parkinson disease: a model for physical therapy. Phys Ther, 80(6), 578–597.

Moyers, P. (1999). Guide to occupational therapy practice. Am J Occupat Ther, 53, 247.

O'Sullivan, S.B. (2001). Strategies to improve motor control and motor learning. In O'Sullivan, S.S. & Schmitz, T.J. (eds.). Physical Rehabilitation: Assessment and Treatment, ed. 4. Philadelphia: F.A. Davis Company.

O'Sullivan, S.B. & Schmitz, T.J. (2001). Physical Rehabilitation Laboratory Manual: Focus on Functional Training. Philadelphia: F.A. Davis Company.

Palmer, M. L. & Toms, J.E. (1992). Manual for Functional Training, ed. 3. Philadelphia: F.A. Davis Company.

Pedretti, L.W. (1996). Occupational Therapy: Practice Skills for Physical Dysfunction, ed. 4. St. Louis: Mosby Company.

Perry, J. (1992). Gait Analysis: Normal and Pathological Function. Thorofare, NJ: Slack, Inc.

Perry, J., Hoffer, M.M., Giovan, P., Antonelli, P. & Greenberg, R. (1986). Predictive value of manual muscle testing and gait analysis in normal ankles by dynamic electromyography. Foot Ankle, 6(5), 254–259.

Pimentel, E.D. (1996). The disappearing reflex: a reevaluation of its role in normal and abnormal development. Phys Occupat Ther Pediatr, 16(4),19–41.

Poole, J. (1997). Movement-related problems. In Christiansen, C. & Baum, C. (eds.). Enabling Function and Well-Being, ed. 2. Thorofare, NJ: Slack, Inc.

Preston, L.A. & Hecht, J.S. (1999). Spasticity Management Rehabilitation Strategies. Bethesda, Md: American Occupational Therapy Association.

Rainville, E.B. (1999). The special vulnerabilities of children and families. In Poor, S.M. & Rainville, E.B. Pediatric Therapy: A Systems Approach. Philadelphia: F.A. Davis Company.

Reed, E. (1982). An outline of a theory of action systems. J Motor Behav, 14, 98–134.

Richards, C.L., Malouin, F., Dumas, F. & Wood-Dauphine, S. (1991). New rehabilitation strategies for the treatment of spastic gait disorders. In Patla, A.E. (ed.). Adaptability of Human Gait: Implications for the Control of Locomotion. New York: Elsevier.

Ryerson, S. & Levit, K. (1997). Functional Movement Reeducation. Philadelphia: Churchill Livingstone.

Schenkman, M.A., Berger, R.A., Riley, P.O., Mann, R.W. & Hodge, W.A. (1990). Whole-body movements during rising to standing from sitting. Phys Ther, 10, 638–651.

Schoen, S. & Anderson, J. (1993). Neurodevelopmental treatment frame of reference. In Kramer, P. & Hinojosa, J. (eds.). Frames of Reference for Pediatric Occupational Therapy. Baltimore: Williams & Wilkins.

Sherlock, J. (1996). Getting into balance. Rehab Manage, Dec/Jan, 33–36.

Shumway-Cook, A. & Woollacott, M.H. (2001). Motor Control: Theory and Practical Applications, ed. 2. Philadelphia: Lippincott Williams & Wilkins.

Sugden, D. A. (1990). Role of proprioception in eye-hand coordination. In Bard, C., Fleury, M., & Hay L. (eds.). Development of Eye-Hand Coordination Across the Life Span. Columbia, SC: University of South Carolina Press.

Tscharnuter, I. (1993). A new therapy approach to movement organization. Phys Occupat Ther Pediatr, 13(2), 19–40.

Umphred, D. (2001). Neurological Rehabilitation, ed. 4. St. Louis: Mosby, Inc.

Umphred, D., Byl, N., Lazaro, R.T. & Roller, M. (2001). Interventions for neurological disabilities. In Neurological Rehabilitation, ed. 4. St. Louis: Mosby, Inc.

Van Sant, A. F. (1990). Life-span development in functional tasks. Phys Ther, 70(12), 788–798.

Verbrugge, L. (1994). The disablement process. Soc Sci Med, 38, 1–14.

Wade, M. & Jones, G. (1997). The role of vision and spatial orientation in the maintenance of posture. Phys Ther, 77(6), 619–627.

World Health Organization. (2001). International Classification of Functioning, Disability, and Health. Geneva, Switzerland: author.